"A MILESTONE IN ORGASMOLOGY!"
—*Publishers Weekly*

"Probably nothing I have written about over the past eight years has generated as much mail as the Coital Alignment Technique."
—"Ask Isadora," *Village Voice*

"Informative, accurate, credible."
—Dr. William Granzig, Chairman, American Board of Sexology, *Atlanta Journal/Constitution*

"In a nation with warnings about safe sex and often fearful of any sex in the age of AIDS, *The Perfect Fit* has come at a perfect time."
—*Reuter's*

"The erotic equivalent of a Monet watercolor ... exciting ... it is actually quite great!"
—*Self*

"Choreographed performance, almost like Astaire and Rogers."
—Dr. Bernie Zilbergeld, author of *The New Male Sexuality*, *New York Newsday*

The Perfect Fit

HOW TO ACHIEVE MUTUAL FULFILLMENT
AND MONOGAMOUS PASSION
THROUGH THE NEW INTERCOURSE

by Edward Eichel
and Philip Nobile

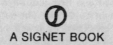

A SIGNET BOOK

SIGNET
Published by the Penguin Group
Penguin Books USA Inc., 375 Hudson Street,
New York, New York 10014, U.S.A.
Penguin Books Ltd, 27 Wrights Lane,
London W8 5TZ, England
Penguin Books Australia Ltd, Ringwood,
Victoria, Australia
Penguin Books Canada Ltd, 10 Alcorn Avenue,
Toronto, Ontario, Canada M4V 3B2
Penguin Books (N.Z.) Ltd, 182–190 Wairau Road,
Auckland 10, New Zealand

Penguin Books Ltd, Registered Offices:
Harmondsworth, Middlesex, England

Published by Signet, an imprint of Dutton Signet,
a division of Penguin Books USA Inc. This is an authorized
reprint of a hardcover edition published by Donald I. Fine, Inc.

First Signet Printing, October, 1993
10 9 8 7 6 5 4 3 2 1

Dedicated to the couples who,
with trust, explored coital alignment.
And to my wife, Joanne,
whose contribution to my work
has been enormous.
—EDWARD EICHEL

To the memory
of Alfred Kinsey.
—PHILIP NOBILE

Contents

Introduction

New sex positions do not grow on trees. From the devout standing postures of Hindu temple maidens to the "X position" popularized in *The Joy of Sex* (1972), erotology seems to have covered the bases. It is probably easier to discover a novel erogenous zone such as women's *fascia d'Albans*, also known as the G spot, than to find an unimagined method of intercourse.

One of the last places to look for innovation in the art of love is the sexology journals that dabble more in exotica like paradigms of desire, pseudohermaphroditism and sexual functioning in kidney transplant patients.

Yet, in the summer of 1988, The Journal of Sex and Marital Therapy, edited by the noted psychiatrist Helen Singer Kaplan, published an article on a new clitoris-friendly technique that performed wonders of orgasm in a study of 86 monogamous men and women.

The title of the astonishingly original paper was "The Technique of Coital Alignment and Its Relation to Female Orgasmic Response and Simultaneous Orgasm." The author was Edward Eichel, a Manhattan psychotherapist and, not surprisingly, something of a maverick in a maverick's profession.

Eichel is a follower of Wilhelm Reich, the Freudian heretic and wild sex genius who created a formula for would-be bigger and better orgasms in the twenties. As a leader of an encounter group in the late sixties in Greenwich Village, Eichel taught couples to make love in the tender style of Reich. There was no watching in his groups; sex was private but the postcoital conversations were very public. However, Eichel added an unusual feature to Reich's orgasm formula. Reich had left the exact position up to the taste and fantasy of the couple. But not Eichel. He developed a technique taking off from the "pelvic override" position in which the man rides high on the woman and presses the base of his penis against her clitoris. Eichel put a spin on the override by substituting a slight rocking and rolling motion for male thrusting, a movement that tended to make the override awkward and uncomfortable for the woman.

Eichel's exciting new technique, which he

titled the Coital Alignment Technique or CAT, elicited strong emotions and orgasms in his encounter group and later among clients in his marriage-therapy practice. Just one in four women in his study climaxed regularly during man-above intercourse before learning the coital alignment, whereas three in four climaxed regularly afterward. The frequency of simultaneous orgasm rose from five to fifty percent with the same women. The technique also seemed to enhance desire for intercourse and the intensity of orgasm in both men and women. When Eichel compared his sample of aligned persons with a matched group untrained in the technique, his people were significantly ahead in every measure of orgasmic satisfaction.

In sum, Eichel's pilot study suggested that Reich's formula, aided by the CAT, produced a higher degree of orgasm, and did so on a steady basis.

In the tradition of Reich, Eichel has gone for the sexual gold. He believes that he has fulfilled his mentor's prophecy by tapping into nature's supposed orgasmic design and that his coital technique is an answer to the age-old dilemma of male-female incompatibility. "It changes the whole concept of sex," he told the Toronto *Sun* in 1989.

No quiet gourmet guide like Alex Comfort, Eichel has warred with the sexology establishment over his technique. "I'm saying that we're operating in this field with a failed model of intercourse and a romanticized model of alternative lifestyles," he told the board of the Society For the Scientific Study of Sex in 1989. "And it is destructive of male-female relating. My research is a breakthrough that can help men and women."

Intercourse and orgasm, as the case of Eichel demonstrates, are risky specialties. The quest for the "perfect fit" became one of the major cultural controversies of the modern era involving the giants of psychoanalysis and sexology as well as an army of amateur investigators. Theories clashed; therapies appeared and disappeared; reputations rose and fell; and even scientific scandal haunted the effort to close the ecstasy gap between men and women. Things became so extreme in the mid-eighties that a Parisian gynecologist started treating the clitorides of non-orgasmic women with *laser* rays.

Edward Eichel's coital alignment is the latest development in the never-ending search for orgasm heaven. In spite of the sexual politics in which it is enmeshed, the CAT will be judged by lovers as time goes by.

I have prefaced an exploration of Eichel's technique and the histories of his beneficiaries with a chapter on the natural history of orgasm, and a chapter on 20th century orgasmology. The first chapter raises primal questions about the sexual differences between men and women. Here I report on recent controversies regarding the clitoris and the penis, and with the help of the Kinsey archives I profile America's orgasmic athletes—gangster men and women who climax from pure fantasy as in Harold Robbins novels. In the second chapter I scrutinize the intercourse and orgasm formulas of towering orgasmologists from Wilhelm Reich to Shere Hite and beyond. And then in the third chapter Edward Eichel has his say and annotates his own illustrated CAT manual. Chapter four consists of Eichel's answers to a series of questions potential CAT users may have. Histories of Eichel's satisfied patients and other admirers of CAT are contained in the fifth and final chapter. The book concludes with an Appendix of tables from Eichel's study in the Human Sexuality Department at New York University assessing the effectiveness of CAT.

A word about the creation of this book: I am the author of the text and had editorial control. Edward Eichel provided instructions for his technique and tapes of his former patients. He also turned over his files and sat for many hours of interviews, for which I am grateful.

Philip Nobile
Scarsdale, N.Y.

CHAPTER 1

A Natural History of Intercourse

A FONDNESS FOR MALE ORGASM

Although the French have no word for it, intercourse is the grand opera of evolution. Except for the odd egg-laying species, all mammals mate the same way—by inserting the penis in the vagina. In the eighteenth century Lord Chesterfield observed that "the position is ridiculous, the pleasure momentary and the expense damnable." Chesterfield was exaggerating. Unless you are a Shaker or Shere Hite, the popularity of intercourse is undeniable. Alfred Kinsey was not a romanticist about sex, yet he rose to the near-lyrical when describing the overarching fantasy that men bring to the main act of love. "The male in many instances may not be having coitus with the immediate sexual partner," he wrote at the close of *Sexual Behavior in the Human Female* (1953), "but with all the other girls with whom he has ever had coitus, and with the entire genus Female with which he would like to have coitus."

Actually, intercourse originates with single-celled protozoans like the amoeba and paramecium. These primitive organisms can reproduce by non-sexual fission for ten thousand generations or more, a proficiency that prompted Charles Darwin to wonder why sexual conjugation developed in the first place. "The whole subject is as yet hidden in darkness," he wrote in 1862 in the *Journal of the Proceedings of the Linneau Society*. But now we know that protozoan cell lines eventually die out in the absence of conjugation whereby two cells hook up and rejuvenate their flagging energy by exchanging vital genetic fluids.

Intercourse does not become blatantly anthropomorphic until mammals appear. Froggy-style rendezvous of urogenital openings, the usual custom of amphibians, are replaced by simple penetration with an exterior male organ. From kangaroo up, reproduction means basic intromission with specialized parts of incongruous shapes and sizes. For examples, the clitorides of some monkeys are longer than the penises of their mates; and the six-hundred-pound male gorilla, the King Kong of primates, has a flaccid phallus less than half the size of that of *Homo sapiens*.

Not surprisingly, mammalian liaisons are fraught with animal tension. Consider cats and dogs. Feline males cannot make entrance without sinking their teeth into the back of the female. In contrast, male canines cannot exit after ejaculation because internal swelling at the base of the penis locks them in. (Could the myth of *vagina dentata* have arisen from Neanderthal man's attempt to understand the post-coital distress of brother dog?)

At the close of a long, distinguished career surveying the creatures of the earth, a legendary British naturalist was asked what single attribute he would ascribe to the Creator? "A fondness for beetles," the old man replied, referring to the fact that beetles rank number one in the fauna population, comprising 350,000 of the 1,250,000 different species that inhabit the planet. If a similar question were posed about what the design of mammalian intercourse implies about the Grand Designer, the answer must be a fondness for male orgasm.

What is almost metaphysical certitude for male mammals—orgasm during intercourse—is generally rare and frequently never for female mammals. Female rabbits seem to exhibit orgasmic movements, as do minks and all members of the cat family. With prolonged masturbation of the clitoral area, captive female monkeys have been moved to climax in the laboratory. But the *Story of O* in the wild is generally for males only. The statistics are better for civilized females, but on any given night millions of them do not climax in coitus.

Where, if at all, has nature gone wrong? The speed factor looks suspicious. Some mammals—lions, horses and skunks—nuzzle in extended foreplay, but copulation itself is typically sudden. Bulls, stallions and rams ejaculate virtually on impact. From start to finish, elephants complete the job in thirty seconds, even though handicapped by an unwieldy five-foot prehensile penis. Minks and sables engage in intercourse for as long as eight hours but our nearest relatives, monkeys and apes, are with the swift majority.

According to a fifty-year-old experiment that timed ninety-five chimpanzee matings, the average insertion was less than ten seconds and involved fewer than twenty thrusts. "It is physically impossible for a male ape to force a female to continue genital contact if she vigorously attempts to escape," wrote Clellan Ford and Frank Beach in *Patterns of Sexual Behavior* (1951). "Therefore, once intromission is achieved, a male who ejaculates quickly has a better chance to fertilize his mate before she terminates the union." And before male competitors or predators start nipping at his heels.

The male trend toward speedy sex endures at the top of the mammalian chain. "In most of the societies for which we have data, it is reported that men take the initiative and, without extended foreplay, proceed vigorously toward climax without much regard for achieving synchrony with the woman's orgasm," wrote anthropologist William Davenport in *Human Sexuality in Four Perspectives* (1976), an anthology edited by Frank Beach.

But who can say with assurance that all that females need is more time to reach climax? Perhaps the problem lies as much or more with the manner of the stimulation than its duration. All mammals save man are restricted to rear entry. Since the genitals of female mammals are located toward the rear, it is the only efficient method. But the clitoris, the most excitable tissue in the pelvic area, is situated above the vagina and remains untouched when consummation is from behind.

Obviously, evolution has been nonchalant about female orgasm. Natural selection paid little attention to responsive females because their climax, unlike the male's, was unnecessary for conception. As a consequence, modern women, it seems, have not uniformly inherited the fittest sexual genes.

In spite of some less than precise thinking

on the topic, Sigmund Freud was correct about the evolutionary cloud hanging over too many boudoirs. In 1935, a Mrs. Springer from Vienna wrote him about her disenchantment with the amatory habits of men. He replied sympathetically, but he put the blame elsewhere:

Dear Madam:

I think that you are right that most men are egotistical and ignorant in their sexual life and don't care enough for the sexual satisfaction of the female. The main fault, however, is yet not on the side of man. Much more of it seems there is a neglect on the side of nature, which is interested only that the purpose of the sexual act is being attained while it shows indifference as to whether the woman gets full satisfaction or not.

The reasons for this strange neglect, about which the female rightfully complains, are not yet recognized with certainty.

Yours very truly,
Freud

Nature has not only neglected female orgasm, it has been capricious in spreading the ability around. Although some women have a sexual nervous system superior to that of the most advanced Don Juan, including the capacity to climax two hundred times in an hour, as well as the knack of "coming" from fantasy alone, a large percent remain ungratified in coitus. The rates of "sexual anesthesia," to recall the quaint nineteenth century term, have varied wildly from sexologist to sexologist. At the beginning of this century the knowing opinion was that the majority of young women were so afflicted. As Dutch physician Th. H. Van de Velde wrote in *Ideal Marriage* (1926), the leading love manual of the day and for years thereafter, "the newly married woman *is as a rule,* more or less completely 'cold' or indifferent to and in sexual intercourse. She must be *taught to love ..."* (emphasis Van de Velde's). But twenty-five years later Kinsey said in his female volume that three-quarters of American brides were orgasmic during intercourse in the first year of marriage and that thirty-nine percent of them were always or almost always so.

Ethnographically speaking, the female orgasm news is bad all over. Dr. Donald Symons, an anthropologist at the University of California at Santa Barbara, summed up the unhappy global situation and noted the shaky status of intercourse in *The Evolution of Human Sexuality* (1979): "Among some peoples female orgasm is unknown; where it is known its occurrence is usually sporadic; in the few societies where all females are said to orgasm, substantial clitoral stimulation occurs during foreplay or during consciously and deliberately prolonged intercourse; orgasm is never considered to be a spontaneous and inevitable occurrence for females as it always is for males. Women's statements about their sensations during intercourse, and the data on masturbation, further undermine the view that women's genitals are designed to generate orgasm during intercourse."

Symons's comment reflected two contradictory views in current orgasmology: (1) the right kind of stimulation can overcome nature's unkindness toward women's coital climax; and (2) intercourse is second-class sexual pleasure, compared to masturbation, and should be knocked off its patriarchal pedestal. Reacting to centuries of oppression, many feminists emphasized the latter. Gloria Steinem's amusing and witty observation that "a woman needs a man like a fish needs a bicycle" was translated into hardcore anti-intercourse polemics. In the *New Our Bodies, Ourselves* (1984), the Boston Women's Health Collective called old-fashioned intromission "a form of lovemaking which is often well-suited to men's orgasm and pleasure but not necessarily well-suited to ours." Shere Hite threw a wrench at the act in *The Hite Report* (1976), when she condemned men for "their almost hysterical fixation on intercourse and orgasm." And the ultra-feminist Andrea

Dworkin went all the way in *Our Blood* (1976), insisting that men, whom she called "prick-proud," will have "to give up their precious erections and begin to make love the way women do together."

This is, it would seem, the viewpoint of some lesbians, but consigning coitus into the dustbin of venereal history is folly, especially since there are ways for unsatisfied women to override evolution and make intercourse an orgasmic occasion. Even Symons noted that coitus worked beautifully for women with the right kind of stimulation. So Eichel's CAT, modeled after Reich's formula, is an idea whose time has arrived, at least as another clitoris-based intercourse position.

THE CLITORIS: TO HAVE AND HAVE NOT

It is no secret that clitoris and penis are anatomical doppelgangers with roughly the same internal and external structures, including nerves, erectile tissue, shaft, foreskin and head. The resemblance goes even to the bone. In those species that retain an abbreviated *os phallus* in the shaft—gorilla, bear, cat and most rodents—there is also a rudimentary piece of bone or gristle in the clitoris. The penis and clitoris not only look alike but also, in spite of some marked differences in size, function and direction (the former points down, the latter up), respond alike during sex.

The main deviation involves the urethral opening. The penis has one and the clitoris does not. "In this sense, women are biologically more evolved as each function [i.e., the sexual and the urinary] has its own orifice," wrote Dr. Thomas Power Lowry in *The Classic Clitoris* (1978). "This female evolutionary advance is further implied by the fact that in men pleasure, reproduction, and urination are united in the penis, while in the woman they are separated in the clitoris, vagina and urethra."

Although female sexuality is a perennial mystery, one need not be a gynecologist to realize that the clitoris, as opposed to the passive vagina, is the seat of female eroticism and the only organ in the human body devoted purely to sexual delight. "Therefore, even the action of the clitoris, which is the female penis, will be erection," noted Francois Plazzoni, a seventeenth century Italian surgeon as quoted by Lowry. "Wanton women themselves admit this erection, inasmuch as they affirm that something in their private parts stiffens and stands out when they are involved in lascivious activity."

Nevertheless, the clitoris, being tiny and seemingly vestigial, has been the object of immense discord from Plazzoni's day to the present. Freud put the enviable piece of flesh back in the limelight in *New Introductory Lectures on Psychoanalysis* (1933), demoting the masculinized clitoris in favor of the more feminine vagina and suggesting that vaginal orgasms were the only healthy way to go:

> . . . in the phallic phase of the girl, the clitoris is the dominant erotogenic zone. But it is not destined to remain so; with the change to femininity, the clitoris must give up to the vagina its sensitivity, and, with it, its importance, either wholly or in part.

According to Freudian dogma, any woman who failed to make this nervous leap was sure to be frigid in intercourse: "In those women who are sexually anaesthetic, as it is called, the clitoris has stubbornly retained this sensitivity," wrote Freud in *A General Introduction to Psychoanalysis* (1935). Since neither Freud nor his followers spelled out *how* to accomplish the switch of erogenous headquarters, women were left in the lurch. Those who could not climax with a penis inside them, even if otherwise orgasmic, were considered somehow disturbed. Karen Horney, one of the first female psychoanalysts, acknowledged feeling a secret shame about her clitoral lust. "I would not for the world admit that this sort of pleasure gives me more satisfaction than the normal sort," Horney wrote in her diary on January 3, 1911.

The notion of vaginal supremacy lingers on. After speaking of "the varsity of sexual achievers" who can climax from nipple stimulation or less, psychiatrist Avidah Offit scapegoated women who were not as orgasmic during intromission. "There is usually some psychological problem, however small or large, when a woman fails to climax with modest frequency during sex [i.e., intercourse] with a competent and likable lover," Dr. Offit stated in her book *Night Thoughts* (1981).

With his characteristic zest for piling up information and solving sexual puzzles, Kinsey got into the clitoris controversy in 1953 with publication of *Sexual Behavior in the Human Female*. As a young entomologist at Harvard, where he earned his doctorate, and at Indiana University, where he was professor of zoology, Kinsey collected four million gall wasps and one-million-and-a-half related insects. When he switched from bugs to sex in the thirties he retained a Darwinian eye for new and fascinating detail. For example, he happened to take the histories of a small cluster of women in rural Kansas who turned out to be one hundred percent orgasmic in intercourse. When he returned to the scene to search for the cause of the anomaly, he noticed that the mothers pacified their infant girls with a particular patting technique that soon induced sleep. "Unbeknownst to the mothers, they were accidentally bringing their baby girls to orgasm, thereby leaving traces in the sexual substrate which made them 'easy responders' for life," recalled Dr. C. A. Tripp, one of Kinsey's colleagues now retired in Nyack, New York, in a conversation with Nobile.[1]

Kinsey was a stickler for the scientific method.[2]

Although he admired Freud for his courage to pursue sex research in a hostile world, he was contemptuous of Freud's sweeping judgments about sex that floated on thin scientific air. For example, he acquired unpublished notes of Freud's early lectures in Vienna and marveled at his disdain for masturbation.

Playing detective with Freud's vaginal-orgasm concept, Kinsey asked five gynecologists (two were female) to measure the genital

[1]Eichel comments: I believe that this anecdotal information, unsupported by a published scientific study, is dangerous. It could be misconstrued by pedophiles as the promotion of sexual contacts with children.

Nobile comments: *All* data on childhood sexuality can be misconstrued by anybody, pedophiles included. But sex researchers cannot exclude such information to prevent worst case scenarios.

[2]Eichel comments: Philip Nobile and I met in relation to my controversial book challenging the early Kinsey research, *Kinsey, Sex and Fraud: The Indoctrination of a People* (1990), co-authored by Dr. Judith A. Reisman, Dr. J. Gordon Muir, M.D., and edited by Dr. John H. Court. Nobile and I have agreed to disagree on this point about Kinsey.

sensitivity of 879 women. The subjects were gently stroked all over the pudenda with a glass, metal or cotton-tipped probe. The clitoris as well as the major and minor lips responded to these touches about ninety-eight percent of the time; in comparison, the vagina was revealed as pretty much a sensory wasteland. Kinsey remarked that vaginal tissue originated embryonically from the egg ducts "which, like nearly all other internal body structures, are poorly supplied with end organs of touch." Only fourteen percent of the women felt the probe inside the vagina and most of them reported sensation on the upper wall close to the vaginal entrance (the site of the alleged G-spot).

Kinsey also applied the masturbation test. Which part did women prefer to rub when onanistically inclined? Kinsey found that the clitoris was preferred over the vagina by better than four to one as a masturbatory site. And even when women inserted fingers into the vagina, the purpose was essentially to get a better grip. Furthermore, wrote Kinsey, lesbians who had "a better than average understanding of female genital anatomy," shunned deep penetration while making love.

Consequently, Kinsey searched in vain for the vaunted vaginal orgasm, concluding that it was a mistake to confuse this psychoanalytic construct with the vaginal spasms that frequently accompany ordinary orgasm. These spasms, he said, were connected with overall bodily convulsions and had nothing to do with the quality of the climax itself.

Except for diehard Freudians, the professor from Indiana University pretty well routed the claim of vaginal orgasm. With mounds of data, Kinsey argued that the clitoris (and surrounding tissue) was the essence of Venus. "No question of 'maturity' seems to be involved," he wrote in the female volume," and there is no evidence that the vagina responds in orgasm as a separate organ . . ."

And what of clitoral size? Kinsey had a question about that on his female questionnaire. But the organ, embedded as it is in fleshy tissue, proved impervious to exact calculations. However, based on unpublished archival data, Kinsey said that black women, like black men, had larger genitals than their Caucasian counterparts. "Clitorises measuring more than an inch are apparently very rare among whites, but may occur in 2 or 3 percent of blacks, or at least they did so in the limited number of black histories we took," Dr. Wardell Pomeroy, Kinsey's co-author, wrote in *Dr. Kinsey and the Institute for Sex Research* (1971). "Long clitorises are well-known among black prostitutes, and measurements of three inches or more were obtained from perhaps one out of 300 or 400 black women."

Masters and Johnson treated Freud's vagina complex as unkindly as Kinsey had. By logging 7,500 orgasms in 382 easily aroused women in the secrecy of their St. Louis lab in the late fifties, they exhaustively explored the action of the clitoris during sex. Their daring landmark research, realized with the help of prostitutes and an electrically powered glass phallus, gained huge notoriety when it was published in *Human Sexual Response* in 1966. Although the couple would subsequently be criticized for inflating their success in treating sex dysfunctions, their early physiological work is considered first rate.

Masters and Johnson advanced the science of the clitoris with two interesting discoveries: (1) the clitoris is slower to erect than the penis and tumescence lags ten to thirty seconds behind vaginal lubrication; (2) as sexual tension increases near orgasm, the head inexplicably retreats under the foreskin and the shaft retracts into the fleshy folds of the mons, losing up to fifty percent of its length. They also confirmed what other sexologists, including Kinsey, had suspected about size and location (the distance from the vaginal opening)— neither factor is related to orgasm.

If the clitoris receded during the high excitement of intercourse, how did it receive enough attention to bestir women to climax? Masters and Johnson thought that, no matter the intercourse position, the thrusting penis exerted indirect pressure on the clitoris by tugging at the swollen minor lips, which in turn pulled down on the clitoral hood, the skin covering the clitoris. Their logic cannot be faulted on this crucial point. After all, their female subjects were having near-clockwork orgasms during traditional in-and-out intercourse (a talent required for participation in the project) and so this penis-to-lips-to-hood-to-clitoris mode of stimulation appeared to be the *only* explanation for coital climax.

Still, there was something missing from Masters and Johnson's picture. As a skeptical Hite pointed out in the first *Hite Report:* "If this mechanism works so well, why hasn't it been working all along, for centuries?" Rejecting Masters and Johnson's model, Hite had an explanation of her own for women's discontent with coitus: "Intercourse was never meant to stimulate women to orgasm," she declared.

Regarding vaginal orgasms, the phantom of psychoanalysis, Masters and Johnson agreed with Kinsey in *Human Sexual Response:* "From an anatomic point of view, there is absolutely no difference in the responses of the pelvic viscera to effective sexual stimulation, regardless of whether the stimulation occurs as a result of clitoral-body or mons-area manipulation, natural or artificial coition, or, for that matter, specific stimulation of any other erogenous area of the female body." In other words, all orgasms are the same.

After Masters and Johnson and the ascendance of feminism, the clitoris was restored to a place of pride in the culture. Reproaching the rosebud was not so much politically incorrect as it was dense. Although the knoll of sexology tends to be grassy with hour-long-orgasm doctors and female-ejaculation boosters, the clitoris was immune from attack until The Journal of Sex Research published an astonishing, anti-zeitgeist paper in the summer of 1989. The article, titled "The Sexual Experience of Marital Adjustment of Genitally Circumcised and Infibulated Females in the Sudan," was the work of Hanny Lightfoot-Klein, an anthropologist, who came back from Africa with the news that the clitoris is overrated over here. She did not regulate it to the appendix class, but declared that her data "seriously question the importance of the clitoris as an organ that must be stimulated in order to produce female orgasm, as is often maintained in Western sexology literature."

She arrived at this opinion after interviewing three hundred women who had undergone the eviscerating Pharaonic circumcision, an ancient Nile Valley rite required of all Moslem females between the ages of four and eight in the desert land of Sudan. Although some African tribes limit excision to the major lips, the Pharaonic type is radical. Operating without anesthesia, untrained midwives remove the clitoris, the minor lips and even the inner layers of the major lips. They finish by infibulating (sewing together) the outer edges of the major lips. The barbaric rite frequently results in hemorrhage, shock and infection as well as mental trauma. When the wound has healed over with "an artificially created chastity belt of thick, fibrous scar tissue," the little girls are left with just a small opening for urination and menstruation. After marriage, penetration is accomplished in pain and sometimes the midwife has to be recalled to slit the opening wider with her knife. Apparently, the victims adjust to their mutilation with stoicism because they believe that it is Allah's will.

What is the masculine logic behind clitoridectomy? Sudan is an unabashed patriarchy—that is, a sexual police state where female chastity is strictly enforced (while young boys are encouraged to try out anal sex with each other). The slightest sexual trespass by a woman can have dire consequences—divorce, exile from the clan and death. "Women are assumed to be (by nature) sexually voracious, promiscuous and unbridled creatures, morally too weak to be entrusted with the sacred honor of the family," explained Lightfoot-

Klein. "Pharaonic circumcision is believed to insure this honor by not only decreasing an excessive sexual sensitivity in them but by considerably dampening their sex drive." This tragic misunderstanding is reinforced by another macabre delusion—an unclipped clitoris will grow larger and hang between a woman's legs.

If genital mutilation were not anaphrodisia enough, Sudanese women suffer further sexual repression: they are forbidden to initiate sex or show delight during intercourse. In contrast to women of the West, they have learned to fake *frigidity*. "If the woman has an orgasm, she hides it, and if she is unable to control the intensity of her reaction, she denies that it was brought on as sexual ecstasy," wrote Lightfoot-Klein.

The anthropologist's findings became more interesting when she described the amazing orgasmic adjustment that her subjects made to their condition. Although climax in women without clitorides is not unknown to sexology, a point that Lightfoot-Klein conceded, she learned that female orgasm is a surprisingly *routine*, though necessarily covert, visitor to the mud huts of the Sudan. "Contrary to expectation, nearly 90% of all women interviewed said that they experienced orgasm (climax) or had at various periods in their marriage experienced it," she wrote. "Frequency ranged from always to rarely. Some women said they had intense, prolonged orgasm, and this was verified by their happy and highly animated demeanor as they described it. Other women said that their orgasms were weak or difficult to achieve."

Here are three accounts of post-circumcision climax quoted by the anthropologist:

All my body begins to tingle. Then I have a shock to my pelvis and my legs. It gets very tight in my vagina. I have a tremendous feeling of pleasure, and cannot move at all. I seem to be flying far, far up. Then my whole body relaxes and I go completely limp.

I feel as if I am losing all my consciousness, and I love him most intently at that moment. I tremble all over. My vagina contracts strongly and I have a feeling of great joy. Then I relax all over, and I am so happy to be alive and to be married to my husband.

I feel shivery and want to swallow him inside my body. Then a very sweet feeling spreads all over my entire body, and I feel as if I am melting. I float higher and higher, far, far away. Then I drift off to sleep.

This degree of pleasure is jarring. Sudanese wives should not feel *that* good with a crippled genital cleft. Lightfoot-Klein speculated that several psychological factors probably compensated for their physical loss: (1) unaware of other cultures, Sudanese women thought all women on earth were circumcised; (2) condemned to the barren and brutal Sahara environment, they were used to living with physical trauma; (3) despite the heartless, antifemale social code, they felt secure in cohesive families and strongly bonded marriages characteristic of the Sudan; and (4) since they are permitted to signal sexual readiness to their husbands by permeating their skin with the smell of burning spices in a ritualized "smoke ceremony," they have *some* emotional command over sexual relations.

Lightfoot-Klein also mentioned the possibility that an erogenous back-up system had kicked in: "Presumably, Pharaonic circumcision also facilitates the enhancement of remaining erogenous zones, and possibly the development of others."

She noted seven documented pathways to female orgasm. Apart from the genitals (clitoris and vagina), she listed breasts, tongue/lips, G-spot, anus and fantasy. When she asked Sudanese women which parts of their body were the most erotically sensitive, they said, in addition to the obvious places, neck, belly, thighs and hips.

Lightfoot-Klein may have uncovered nothing new in Africa, except that a whole tribe of mutilated women managed to have regular coital climax without resort to the rosebud.

But even this claim is in doubt, owing to the imprecision of her data.

For example, she did not disclose the exact numbers behind the orgasmic frequency of her subjects. It does not mean a great deal to say that ninety percent of the Sudanese women had at least a *single* orgasm in their lives if the actual rate of occurrence is undefined. When she wrote that frequency ranged between always and rarely, she should have provided a breakdown. What if only ten percent had orgasm every time and ninety percent were in the rare category?

The second difficulty would seem more serious: not once did the anthropologist define orgasm, the very item she was testing. Granted the language barrier and the clash of cultures, how could she be sure that she and her subjects were talking about the same phenomenon? Sex is an immensely intimate and idiosyncratic enterprise. Orgasm, however, is not. Either you have one or you do not. The accepted definition is from Kinsey's male volume: orgasm is "the explosive discharge of neuromuscular tensions at the peak of sexual response." Orgasm cannot be "verified" by merely recording the "happy and highly animated demeanor" of interviewees describing their supposed peaks.

"It's an amateur study by an untrained observer using do-it-yourself criteria," said Dr. C.

A. Tripp, a former protégé of Kinsey's and author of *The Homosexual Matrix* (1975), after reading Lightfoot-Klein's article in The Journal of Sex Research. "If I follow her argument, circumcised Sudanese women have a sex life rivaling that of American women in desire, pleasure and orgasm. And I just can't accept that." Tripp's skepticism is understandable. Quite apart from clitoridectomy, Lightfoot-Klein would have us believe that the condition of psychosexual torture among Sudanese women, a mild form of which has reputedly frozen generations of their counterparts in the West, has no negative effects on sexual response.

But even if she were correct about the bliss of her mutilated subjects, her discovery would not indicate a rewrite of the sex texts, which have already noted the existence of the clitoral bypass. After all, what conceivable lesson can the clitoral have-nots teach the haves? Not to cultivate their most arousing part? Lightfoot-Klein, like many sex researchers, has stretched her case. Her trek into the dark continent of Pharaonic circumcision is far more relevant to anthropology, perhaps, than sexology.

THE PENIS: A MARVEL

The penis is a physiological marvel, too, a true Venice of arteries and caverns that can

double its size at the slightest provocation—
from hearing the national anthem to seeing
one's name in print. "The change between
flaccidity and rigidity in the penis is . . . a tri-
umph of bio-mechanism that no engineer
would have thought possible," observed Dr.
Robert L. Dickinson, a pioneering American
sexologist, in the *Atlas of Human Sex Anatomy*
(1933). "It provides for a powerful tension
that is prolonged yet not painful, by means of
a perfectly balanced inrush and outflow of
fluid, and it also permits semen to pass while
effectively shutting off the bladder contents;
furthermore it plans for six major glands to
cooperate in orderly rhythm and progression."

Compared to other primates, the human
male is extraordinarily well endowed, dwarf-
ing monkeys, gorillas and chimps in both the
penis and testicle department. What was
the species advantage for having the biggest
sex organs? It could not be for aggressive display, because human behemoths can have
small penises and Napoleon-types gargantuan
ones.[3] Or for sexual display because women in

[3]As regards Napoleon, a letter to the *New York Times Book Review*
(August 18, 1991) mentioned that his penis did not go to the grave with
him: "Napoleon's penis was removed from his body by the surgeons
attending him at his death. The penis eventually came on the market
with other relics from the estate of Abbé Ange Paul Vignali, Napoleon's
chaplain on St. Helena, and was offered by the Rosenbach Company in
a 1924 catalogue where it was item No. 9—described as "a mummified
tendon taken from Napoleon's body during the post-mortem." The penis
then found its way into a prominent New Jersey collection and is now
owned by a surgeon at the Columbia Presbyterian Medical Center.

massive numbers do not appear to prize the *membrum virile* over other manly parts. Or to facilitate copulatory success, because there is no evidence indicating that women as a class vastly prefer the brotherhood of the long pole.

In *Sperm Competition and the Evolution of Animal Mating Systems* (1984), biologist Robert Smith proposed a more practical reason for man's superior length: "delivery of ejaculate as close as possible to ova ... a substantially shorter (than optimal) penis would obviously place its owner's ejaculates at a disadvantage in competition with those deposited by a longer organ."

Art, almost an exclusively male province in history, has imitated evolution. The pornography of every known society, except China, magnifies the phallic dimensions. Even Shakespeare granted homage to size in *Antony and Cleopatra*. In the first act, two of Cleopatra's women-in-waiting consult a soothsayer who prophesies similar fortunes for them both.

"Am I not an inch of fortune better than she?" wonders one woman.

"Well, if you were but an inch of fortune better than I," the other says, "where would you choose it?"

"Not in my husband's nose," comes the reply.

The male anatomical obsession that will not die reappeared with a vengeance in Clarence

Thomas v. Long Dong Silver, which was argued last fall on national television. So, like it or not, men are prisoners of size, and from long ago. The *Kama Sutra*, the fifth century B.C. manual of Hindu eroticism, divided men into hares, bulls and stallions according to the length of their *lingam*. A hundred years later Hippocrates insulted the Scythians for their allegedly midget genitals. But it was not until the nineteenth century that cross-cultural penis measurement went semiscientific. Comparisons between blacks and whites, and sometimes Asians, are rooted in the tracts of colonial doctors, explorers and anthropologists of the eighteenth and nineteenth centuries. Sir Richard Burton (1821–90), the libertine British adventurer and prolific litterateur, observed in his translation of *The Arabian Nights* that: "Debauched women prefer Negroes on account of the size of their parts. I measured one man in Somaliland who, when quiescent, numbered nearly six inches. This is characteristic of the Negro race and of African animals (e.g., the horse) . . ."

The primary tome on penis and race is *Wanderings in the Untrodden Fields of Anthropology* (1895) by French army surgeon Jacobus Sutor. Inquisitive about the size, shape, color and smell of male and female organs, Sutor toured the French colonies in Africa, the Near East and Asia gathering information. "I do not deem it more shameful and disgusting to measure the length, the size or the stiffness in erection of a Negro's penis than it would be for a surgeon to probe a urethra, or perform an operation on a testicle," he wrote, justifying his peculiar project. After reviewing this bizarre literature in *Machines As the Measure of Man* (1989), Rutgers University historian Michael Adas concluded that the contents were relentlessly racist: "In virtually all ways, from the shape of their skulls to the size of their penises, Africans more closely resembled apes than Europeans." (Actually, the ape analogy is off because they are the Sycthians of the jungle.)

Hoping to defuse male preoccupation with measurement, modern sexologists tend to dismiss discussion of penis size altogether. "Sex counselors who aren't and don't wish to appear unsympathetic are just about fed up with answering anxious people's questions about penile size," says Dr. Alex Comfort in *The Joy of Sex*. "We've spent years telling enquirers, correctly, that penile size is, functionally, wholly unimportant, that most people who worry that they are smaller aren't . . . that the *only difference* between penises which are large and small when flaccid, a few rare conditions excepted, is that the large kind enlarge less on erection" (emphasis added).

If Comfort really means that in erection all

men's penises are essentially alike in length and circumference, then his erotic egalitarianism betrays common sense. It is inconceivable that erect penises forbid individual variations in size.

Dr. William Masters and Virginia Johnson knew better. After studying the measurements of eighty subjects, they stated in *Human Sexual Response* that "the smaller penis in the flaccid state usually remains somewhat smaller in the erect state." Although Masters and Johnson scrupulously avoided revealing measurement in inches, the few figures mentioned in *Human Sexual Response*—always with the fig leaf of centimeters—permit the reader to make his or her own calculations. The average difference between the small and large flaccid penis is two centimeters or .78 inch in erection.

Even so, Masters and Johnson evaded the question of comparative *length of erection* by shifting the focus to *the measure of increase*. "The difference in average erective size increase between the smaller flaccid penis and the larger flaccid penis is not significant." In the end there is still a .78-inch difference that Masters and Johnson did not address.

Uncharacteristically squeamish about penis size, they have withheld their own findings. "Measurements were done, but we decided not to publicize them at all," Dr. Masters admitted in a Playboy interview (November

1979). "Some damn fools have publicized measurements somewhere." In defense of this silence, he said that knowledge of data on the length of the penis would lead men to the measuring stick. "That way lies impotence."

"It isn't scientific," Virginia Johnson added. "We have more of a commitment to prevention than to the pure science information."

According to politically correct sexology, the races are presumed equal below the belt. Even Swedish sociologist Gunnar Myrdal deemed it necessary to deny genital discrimination in his historic *An American Dilemma: The Negro Problem in Modern Democracy* (1944), which shook the foundations of Southern apartheid in the forties. Liberal sexologists followed this line without presenting supporting data. "Contrary to some widely accepted myths, the size of the penis is not related to a man's body build, skin color, or sexual prowess," Dr. Erwin Haeberle declared in *The Sex Atlas* (1978).

The penis-length "coverup" continues in the present. Dr. June Reinisch, the embattled director of the Kinsey Institute, sits on the largest collection of measurements in the world outside of Czechoslovakia (where sex researcher Jan Raboch acquired twenty thousand sets from army recruits), yet she has not released exact figures.

What was a joke to Shakespeare is no joke

to Dr. Reinisch. According to the mail from the men who read her syndicated column, their biggest sexual worry, after how to gain and maintain an erection, is penis size. Her correspondents are desperate to learn if they are over or under the average.

So it made sense that Dr. Reinisch would include a question about this confounding private part on the National Sex Knowledge Test, which provided the opening chapter of her book entitled *The Kinsey Institute New Report on Sex: What You Must Know To Be Sexually Literate* (1990). However, Dr. Reinisch arranged the answer to the touchiest question on the test—about erection length—so as to avoid upsetting the male bourgeoisie.

The 1,974 "representative Americans" who took the test prior to publication faced an array of choices when asked:

What do you think is the length of an average man's *erect* penis?

a. 2 inches	e. 6 inches	i. 10 inches
b. 3 inches	f. 7 inches	j. 11 inches
c. 4 inches	g. 8 inches	k. 12 inches
d. 5 inches	h. 9 inches	l. Don't know

Reinisch allowed for three correct responses (d, e, f), claiming that the average erection is five inches, six inches and seven inches.

What at first might seem a scientific impossibility was explained a few pages later when Reinisch elaborated on the answers. She cited Kinsey and sexologist John Money as her sources for the three-inch range. "The Kinsey Research as well as an analysis of data by John Money indicate that the average erect penis measures five to seven inches in length," she wrote. In fact, Kinsey and Money said nothing of the kind. "During the process of writing this book, accuracy and sensitivity have been my main objectives," Reinisch stated in the preface. On the subject of erection, she sacrificed the latter for the former.

According to Kinsey's penis data, buried in the Institute's files for almost thirty years, the correct answer to the average erection question was extremely controversial. This was not because Kinsey unearthed something shocking—his data were similar to the few extant penis-length studies—but because his figures were segregated into black and white samples (just as he divided his histories according to age, religion, gender and other classifications). Rather than discuss these ticklish specifics, however, Reinisch went with the safer five-to-seven-inch range.

Indeed, Kinsey's penis statistics are among the best-kept secrets of sexology. Fascinated by sex variations, Kinsey and his team interviewed about twenty-five hundred white college and non-college men, along with fifty-nine college blacks, who sent back four self-administered measurements (length and circumference in the flaccid and erect states). Too arcane for the male report in 1948, this news was not published until 1979 in *The Kinsey Data: Marginal Tabulations of the 1938–1963 Interviews Conducted by the Kinsey Institute for Sex Research.* The results, which favor black men in every dimension, have generally been ignored.

A reader needs to be a mathematical savant to obtain racial averages from reading the penis tables in *Kinsey Data* because they are arranged to show only what percent of the black and white samples is found at quarter-inch intervals from one inch to over ten inches. But in 1983, at the request of Money, the Institute converted the percentages and provided the separate averages for both blacks and whites. Money, a grand old man of the field as well as Reinisch's mentor, cited them in a paper on micropenises (averaging between one and two inches erect) published in the Journal of Sex and Marital Therapy in 1984. He disclosed for the first time in a scientific journal that the myth was true: on average, black men have longer erections than whites by a relatively thin margin of 6.44 inches to 6.13 inches. Despite the pedigree of this information, Reinisch decided that American males would sleep better in ignorance.

Reinisch's unscientific posture, more characteristic of a media therapist than a successor to Kinsey, has landed her in trouble with authorities at Indiana University where the Kinsey Institute is housed. In 1988, six years into her directorship, IU demanded her resignation, accusing her of poor scholarship and mismanagement. Among the many charges contained in a confidential report by the faculty review committee was that Reinisch wasted too much time and money on public relations: ". . . Indiana University should not resort to an effort to emulate Dr. Ruth."

"We used the range in inches because it's the appropriate number," attested Reinisch on the telephone from her office on the Bloomington campus of Indiana University. "When I answer questions about sex, I feel very strongly that I have to always keep in mind a person alone and frightened. People feel anxiety and pain, which causes them to write us. I want to reassure them. So if you say that the average erection is six inches, half the men below will be upset. It's a judgment that I made."

As for the black-white differences, Reinisch stayed clear of them, she said, because she did not trust Kinsey's fifty-nine-man black sample: "I don't feel there's enough data yet to support the black figures."

It may seem unfair to judge black men from such a scanty group. But the laws of statistics permit surveying a relatively small number when the variation tested is also small. Wardell Pomeroy, who labored alongside Kinsey for thirteen years, told Nobile that since the vast majority of measured penises (i.e., eighty-five percent) fall within one inch of the average, fifty-nine blacks suffice to compute average penis length. Increasing the sample size would not improve the accuracy of the result. For example, Kinsey broke his white sample down between 2,376 college whites and 143 non-college whites. And when he compared the length of erection of each group, the figures were virtually identical—6.12 vs. 6.14.

Actually, Kinsey's data show more pronounced racial contrasts in flaccidity, where blacks have an average length of 4.34 inches compared to 3.84 inches for whites, almost a half-inch difference. As for circumference, the average is 3.78 inches for blacks and 3.16 for whites, which represents slightly more than a half-inch discrepancy.

Yet in erection the disparity almost disappears, not even measuring up to Shakespeare's "inch of fortune" in either length or circumference. For instance, the erection gap is only

.31 inches, which is less than 1/18th of the whole span. As for erect circumference, the divergence is only .13 of an inch (4.96 for blacks vs. 4.83 for whites). Nevertheless, even tiny phallic differences loom large in the minds of Iron Johns.

If the penis tends to be a taboo item in America, bones are not. Last fall, when the *Dallas Morning Herald* (October 8, 1991) broke a story saying that Afro-American astronauts might have an advantage on extended space missions because of their greater bone density (bones tend to lose strength during prolonged weightlessness), it did not incite national concern. (Incidentally NASA disassociated itself from the research on which the claims were based.) But a white society that has historically and incorrectly regarded blacks as sexually out of control will probably never be relaxed about exploring black eroticism for its own sake and significance.

Since physical fetishism is not a common female trait, penile proportions concern men far more than women. The annals of sex research appear bare of women's preferences in this area. Hite tried to fill the vacuum by asking women in her first report if penile dimension made a difference: "What shape and size do you find are most compatible with your body—long and fat, short and fat, long and thin, etc." The responses were scanty.

Hite perhaps did not pursue the issue with women because of personal conviction. "Happily, penis size has nothing to do with whether or not women orgasm during intercourse," she observed later in *The Hite Report on Male Sexuality* (1981), though without providing substantial back-up data. However, in the same book, based on questionnaires from 7,180 American men, she confirmed that the majority of phallus owners "wished over and over again that their penis could be just a little larger."

Though some women have an undeniable taste for men who could make love to the Lincoln Tunnel, most seem to accept more modest proportions. And since Kinsey found that only two percent of American men have erections greater than eight inches (blacks were somewhat superior in this category, too), aficionados of size would not have a huge pool to choose from in any case. To put it simply: it's not the meat but the motion, not the wand but the magician.

This sentiment is in accord with the dynamics of female orgasm, which depends on clitoral stimulation supplied by the *base* of the penis, where all men are, after all, practically equal.

THE PERFECT FIT

ATHLETES OF ORGASM

The late mythologist Joseph Campbell told Bill Moyers during "The Power of Myth" PBS series that evolution is basically meaningless—nothing more than "protoplasm reproducing itself." Or in the words of Gore Vidal in *The Nation* (October 28, 1991): "Men and women are dispensable carriers, respectively, of seeds and eggs; programmed to mate and die, mate and die, mate and die." The good news is that the blind instinct for intercourse flourishes at the top of the mammalian scale. While the reproductive activities of four-legged animals are confined to brief periods of female heat, every day is a potential honeymoon for primates like us who are ungoverned by periodic secretions.

Man-above is the most fashionable coital position around the world according to Clellan Ford and Frank Beach. In Polynesia, where the prone Western-style was baptized the "missionary" position, a man squats or kneels over the woman whose legs straddle his thighs. Woman-above, reputedly the best for arousing the clitoris, tends to be in second place most everywhere. But this was not always so. Kinsey learned that less than a third of American women occasionally sat on their lovers, whereas the women of ancient Greece and Rome did so most of the time. "The position with the female above is similarly the commonest in the ancient art of Peru, India, China, Japan and other civilizations," he wrote in *Sexual Behavior in the Human Male* (1948).

Although *homo sapiens* has descended from a long line of seasonal breeders, he has picked up the pace of intercourse in his two hundred thousand years of life on earth. Here is Charles Darwin's description of the sexual supermen of evolution from *The Descent of Man and Selection in Relation to Sex* (1871):

There can be little doubt that the greater size and strength of man, in comparison with woman, together with his broader shoulders, more developed muscles, rugged outline of body, his greater courage and pugnacity, are all due in chief part to inheritance from his half-human male ancestors. These characteristics would, however, have been preserved or even augmented during the long ages of man's savagery, by the success of the strongest and boldest men, both in the general struggle for life and in their contest for wives; a success which would have ensured their leaving a more numerous progeny than their less favoured brethren.

Getting matters going early, nature has lavished some preadolescent males with the sexual strength of lions. Kinsey found that half of a special sample of 182 boys under the age of fourteen were able to achieve two orgasms in rapid succession and that thirty percent could have five or more fairly quickly. These data were obtained, Kinsey explained, from scientifically trained persons, some of them pedophiles, who kept records of their sexual observations or encounters with children.[4] En route to puberty, boys are doused in testosterone, nature's love potion. As their genitalia mature and daily production of spermatozoa rises beyond the seventy million mark, they feel a mammalian rush. "More than 99 percent of the boys begin regular sex lives immediately after the first ejaculation," wrote Kinsey in the male volume, noting that the male *capacity* for repeated orgasms peaks prior to adolescence, though *actual performance* peaks in the middle to late teen years.

Like Darwin, Kinsey believed that men are generally called to coital glory, though relatively few are chosen, owing to various genetic and cultural factors. If a man fell to earth in the fabulously eroticized Mangaian tribe on the Cook Islands of Polynesia, he would be taught to have frequent and vigorous intercourse and he would be judged for his skills in inducing multiorgasm in a variety of part-

[4]In *Kinsey, Sex and Fraud* (1990), Reisman, Eichel, and Muir objected to Kinsey's use of this information from pedophile data. Nobile reviewed their book in the December 11, 1990, *Village Voice.*

ners. On the other end of the spectrum, the men of Inis Beag, a pseudonymous rural village in Ireland studied by anthropologist William Davenport, have almost no intercourse at all. Discouraged from engaging in "shameful" activities, they do not marry until their mid-thirties. The sexual climate is so inclement in Inis Beag, observed Davenport in *Four Perspectives,* that "even the ability of women to experience orgasm is denied, or if admitted, it is considered to be deviant."

But Kinsey was convinced that American men and women, left to their own uncivilized desires, would have considerably more sex than they were accustomed to. Kinsey was biased in favor of action, the more the better. His let-the-feast-begin outlook was expressed between the lines and sometimes popped up in the text. For instance, this comment from the female volume: "... considering the physiology of sexual response and the mammalian backgrounds of human behavior, it is not so difficult to explain why a human animal does a particular thing sexually. It is more difficult to explain why each and every individual is not involved in every type of sexual activity."

"People who criticize Kinsey for cheering on sex in any form are correct," said his old friend Tripp. "He reveled in all kinds of sexual action and looked askance at whatever blocked it. You see his attitude in his interview technique, where he deliberately assumed that the subject had done whatever he asked about. This was useful in squeezing out information that otherwise might have been covered up."

Kinsey was an apple-a-day advocate: "It seems safe to assume that daily orgasm would be in the capacity of the average human male, and that the more than daily rates which have been observed for some primate species could be matched by a large portion of the human population if sexual activity were unrestricted," he wrote in his male volume. "The males who are astounded to find out that 7.6 percent of the population does, in actuality, have daily or more than daily outlet are, in most cases, simply unaware of their own capacities. Since this percentage of males already has daily rates, in spite of the restrictions on their behavior, it is probable that such a percentage of the population would, under optimal conditions, be involved in still more frequent activity."

Whence this athleticism? Possibly men have inherited a reserve of sexual energy from select forebears like the ruminants (deer, camels, cattle, sheep) that have harems to satisfy and are thus constantly rearoused in the presence of new females. This widespread mammalian phenomenon is called the Coolidge Effect, after Calvin Coolidge.

The official version—though sounding apocryphal—was rendered by Dr. G. Bermant in *Psychological Research: the Inside Story* (1976), an anthology edited by M.H. Siegel and H.P. Zeigler:

> One day the President and Mrs. Coolidge were visiting a government farm. Soon after their arrival they were taken off on separate tours. When Mrs. Coolidge passed the chicken pens she paused to ask the man in charge if the rooster copulates more than once each day. "Dozens of times" was the reply. "Please tell that to the President," Mrs. Coolidge requested. When the President passed the pens and was told about the rooster, he asked, "Same hen every time?" "Oh, no, Mr. President, a different one each time." The President nodded slowly, then said "Tell that to Mrs. Coolidge."

Animal experts noticed what became known as the Coolidge Effect when they compared the mating habits of captive bulls and rams with their amatory behavior in the wild. For example, when a bull consummates with a cow under laboratory conditions, sometimes ejaculating as many as eighteen times in a single session, he loses all erotic interest in her afterward. Nothing, it seems, can prod the bull into recoupling with his previous partner. However, this postcoital disinterest is not what it seems. Actually, when a bull has access to a number of different estrous cows on the farm, he becomes insatiable. As long as a new female is introduced each time, the bull can last and last. Science has not yet tested the sexual limits of ruminants at the orgy, though rams are known to have as many orgasms with the twelfth ewe as with the first.

Since most males of our species have no need for quick communions with a series of fresh females, the Coolidge Effect has not flowered among humans. But there are small hints of vestigial CE. First, true male multiple orgasm—two or more ejaculations off the same erection *without a refractory period*—is an oddity except for the precocious preadolescents. Yet Kinsey found that fifteen to twenty percent of males in their teens and early twenties are capable of having several climaxes in a matter of minutes or hours, an ability that still remains in three percent of men in their sixties.

Second, everybody knows that men have an irrepressible yearning for a variety of partners. But nobody knew until Kinsey that extramarital sex is the only sexual outlet that does not decline with age, indicating that diversity is the greatest aphrodisiac for men, as it is for bulls.

Some men, of course, are more athletic than others, prompting the question, are Casanovas born or made? "The simple answer is both," said Tripp. "They have an unusual capacity to get aroused to the point of orgasm by whatever means, owing to an extraordinarily robust sexual substrate—that is, all the nerves, muscles, reflexes, glands, and even psychological input involved in sex. However, I believe that a platform response—an early frustration that creates a lifetime craving that can never be fulfilled—is necessary for maximum outlet. A platform response is always psychological and the product of learning."

Tripp's paradigm for platform response is a certain European gentleman, a minor nobleman as well as a concentration camp survivor, who has recorded over twenty-five thousand sexual episodes since 1950. In 1980, at the age of sixty-eight, he allegedly had sex with thirteen hundred different men while living in India. His history, consisting of charts, diaries and letters, was one of the treasures of the Kinsey archives until it was lost some time in the seventies. As Tripp explained, when the nobleman was a young boy he yearned to be with the male peasants who worked the family estate but his father forbade such contact. Apparently the force of this repression was deeply felt and the nobleman developed an unquenchable appetite for men of the so-called lower social classes.

Kinsey identified gangsters as the most orgasmic class of American men. Among their predilections was a taste for standing intercourse. Although Kinsey did not live to read Mario Puzo's *The Godfather*, he would, one ventures, have appreciated the authenticity of the fictional and hypersexed Sonny Corleone. (What moviegoer does not recall the wedding scene when Sonny made love vertically with one of the bridesmaids?)

Although Kinsey commented only briefly on his criminal contingent, a computer search of unpublished Kinsey data on this special group reveals arresting features of underworld sex practices, including the fact that almost two-thirds of the gangsters had premarital intercourse in the standing position as opposed to twenty-five percent of the college population.

How did Kinsey come to interview these wanted men? He was interested in the sexual patterns of all kinds of people. Criminals constituted one of the seven occupation categories used in the male volume. In the course of his journey through the demimonde, Kinsey met eighty-one bootleggers, con men, dope peddlers, gamblers, hold-up men, pimps, prostitutes and Mafia types, and sat them down to his standard questionnaire involving three hundred to five hundred items (e.g., does seeing yourself nude in the mirror arouse you sexually? What was the greatest number of times you had intercourse in any one week?).

The eighty-one cases represented less than two percent of the overall sample of fifty-three hundred men. But Kinsey could not fail to note the preeminence of criminals in his high-frequency histories, in which the minimum performance was seven orgasms a week. Compared to the six other occupational groups the criminals had the largest percent of high-frequency intercourse. Half of the outlaws (forty of eighty-one) found themselves in this stratospheric region. Semi-skilled laborers followed with just sixteen percent.

Kinsey was obviously impressed by the extraordinary frequency of sex in the underworld. Since only 7.6 percent of all American men had orgasms daily, the fifty percent high-frequency ranking of the criminals suggested a significant sexual difference between the bad guys and the good guys.

How unrestrained were these super-sexual criminals? Consider the number of premarital coital partners: half of the criminals (fifty-two percent) had more than fifty partners before marriage, compared to nine percent of Kinsey's non-college sample and three percent of his college population. This monumental distinction shows that criminals are indeed a class apart.

The tables in *Kinsey Data* contrast the attitudes and practices of college and non-college populations. Here Kinsey's criminals are compared with non-college men in the main because the differences with college types were too pronounced.

Here are the statistics of the sociopathic Don Juans:

- two-thirds of the criminals began masturbating before puberty, compared to one-third of the non-college men;
- twice as many criminals as non-college men had "much" cunnilingus in their first marriage;
- twice as many criminals as non-college men experienced "much" fellatio in their first marriage;
- thirty-five percent of the married criminals had sex with prostitutes, compared to fifteen percent of the non-college men;
- sixty-eight percent of the criminals were fellated by prostitutes, compared to forty-nine percent of the non-college men;
- eighty-six percent of the criminals had some homosexual experience after puberty, compared to forty percent of the non-college men;
- sixty-nine percent of the criminals had extensive homosexual experience, that is, more than fifty-one times and with more than

twenty-one partners, compared to thirteen percent of the non-college men;

* seventeen percent of the criminals disapproved of homosexuality, compared to fifty-five percent of the non-college men. (This taste for homosexual activities is part of the omni-erotic criminal pattern—anything goes.)

Kinsey saluted the goodfellas when he said that ordinary people would be more sexually active if they had criminal minds ever-ready to defy law and custom. He meant that high arousal feeds off violation—e.g., seducing a virgin, stalking thy neighbor's wife, etc.—and criminals have made violation a way of life.

What about the woman's equivalent of a Sonny Corleone? Novelist Harold Robbins has portrayed the female athlete at play in memorably bold scenes, such as in *Memories of Another Day* (1979), in which two strangers meet for the first time in the dining car of a cross-country train and the woman declares "I just came" after being propositioned by the man.

"Ten percent of females have a sexual response equal to or greater than the male response," Tripp commented to Nobile. Of that group, seven out of ten are more or less indistinguishable from males in frequency, ease of arousal and so forth. But three of the ten are far in excess. They can do things that no male can do. For example, sit in a chair, not move a muscle and on command come to orgasm by fantasy alone. No male can do that. They can, in effect, masturbate to orgasm without touching themselves. These highly responsive women are not necessarily high-outlet because they might be rigidly religious or married to men who often say no.

Tripp was referring to Kinsey's sample of seventy-four fantasists who were barely mentioned in the female report. Like the Robbins character, they can proceed to orgasm without moving a muscle. The average time from start to climax was nine minutes—one did it in less than two.

A computer search for these supreme cases shows that fifty-two of them reached climax by other masturbatory methods as well, but twenty-two had orgasms *only* by wishing them. Who *were* these women? Did they climax around the clock? Were they precocious in sex? Promiscuous as adults? Happily married? Did they get along with their parents? Go to church?

At first glance Kinsey's fantasists were not very unusual. "We were never able to predict these women," Pomeroy said in an interview with Nobile. "There was nothing obviously different about them. They weren't sexier looking."

In fact, the fantasists were average women

in most respects. They represented the full array of society—criminals, housewives and upper-class professionals. There were fifty-two Protestants, thirteen Jews, four Catholics and only one without expressed religious preference. Although more than half were not ardent worshippers, one in five considered herself very devout. Three-quarters had fair to good relationships with their fathers. As a group, they did not dance, smoke or play cards more than ordinary women. But many of the fantasists threw themselves into these leisure pursuits with abandon, reflecting a far greater attraction for fun and games.

For example, a third of the fantasists were enthusiastic dancers, yet merely two percent of Kinsey's general sample swayed with music regularly. Twenty percent of the fantasists smoked a pack of cigarettes a day, compared to two percent of the rest. Card-playing regularly occupied a third of the fantasists, but not even one percent of the rest cut the deck frequently.

Given the physical nature of orgasm, women with this finely tuned sensitivity should be biologically distinct. Nevertheless, their sexual development seems entirely normal, that is, they did not mature any differently from average women in terms of age of puberty, menarche, first appearance of pubic hair and breast development. Nor did the fantasists have relatively more sex at early ages. For instance, only two of the women had intercourse before thirteen. As for physical masturbation, the frequency of the fantasists was approximately the same as for the general population.

Despite a high sex drive, these women were less than nymphomaniacal. Almost two-thirds had three or fewer lovers before marriage. And only eight of the twenty-nine married women engaged in extramarital affairs.

One difference appeared significant. The fantasists were more than twice as likely to be college educated. Dr. Paul Gebhard, another co-author of the Kinsey Reports and the former director of the Kinsey Institute, recalled for Nobile that two of the fantasists who demonstrated their orgasmic powers for Kinsey were professional types. Dr. Gebhard believes that education itself is a powerful factor in female sexuality. "We took the histories of a group of career women who belonged to a business club in New York City," he said on the telephone from his retirement home near the Kinsey Institute in Bloomington, Indiana. "Sexually speaking, they were extraordinary. They were intelligent, aggressive and very responsive—a high percentage were multi-orgasmic. If they wanted something, they went after it."

Neither Pomeroy nor Gebhard could explain why their boss heaped superlatives on the fantasists. Although Kinsey insisted that these women responded more quickly, intensely and with more frequent orgasms than men, the evidence does not clearly prove the claim.

However, there is at least one item in the data that dramatically supports Kinsey's point. While merely six percent of his male sample showed "definite and/or frequent arousal" when viewing Hollywood films of the thirties and forties, twenty percent of the fantasizing females were excited by the same scenes.

The fact that fantasists were not promiscuous is a puzzle. Whenever extremes show up in male development, high sexual outlet tends to follow. For instance, boys who arrive at puberty early masturbate sooner and more often and have more sex throughout their lives than more slowly maturing males. Multi-orgasmic men likewise have more sex than ordinary fellows and constitute thirty percent of Kinsey's high-frequency sample—although they are only ten percent of the male population at age twenty-five.

Why don't female fantasists move around the erogenous zones with greater vigor? Pomeroy offered a clue when he mentioned that female capacity for orgasm and performance are not necessarily related. "We knew a woman who could be walking down the street, rub her shoulder against a companion and have an orgasm in broad daylight," he told Nobile. "Yet that same woman would go the next two years without another climax." Pomeroy cited an equally unusual woman in his Kinsey biography. She was a sixty-year-old who could have twenty orgasms in twenty minutes, but was completely frigid before the age of forty.

Gebhard ventures the opinion that men may be just as talented as women in the realm of fantasy orgasms, but opt for the simpler hands-on approach. "However, if some men were truly sex-starved and wanted to fantasize to orgasm, I believe we would see more of it."

Kinsey did not suggest that females, if they would only get into the swing, would have daily sex, too. He did not have to. Anatomically, women are perfectly suited to repeatedly pleasing congress: they do not depend on erection and their orgasms are not as exhausting because there are no glands to refill. As Kinsey pointed out in the female volume, women hold all the orgasm records in premarital petting, masturbation and coitus, not to mention pure fantasy. Nevertheless, despite a generally superior physical capacity for climax, women are the second gender in terms of raw desire and aggression. This psychological difference shows up in nocturnal orgasm, the only category, Kinsey noted in the female volume, in which "maximum frequencies for the females fall below the maximum frequency for the males." Even his fantastic two percent, who came from just thinking, lagged behind the top-ranked male dreamers.

Camille Paglia, bisexual author of *Sexual Personae* (1990) and anti-feminist provocateur, recently declared that on the whole her gender does not play the erotic game with the same élan as the boys. Here is some frank confession between the always subversive Paglia and Susie Bright, former editor of the lesbian magazine *On Our Backs,* as published in *NYQ* (November 10, 1991), a gay weekly magazine published in New York City:

SB: But at this point there's got to be more to why you're not having this wild sex life than lack of opportunity. You're not going to be able to use that as an excuse anymore.

CP: Well, at this point, no, because there are star fuckers and groupies, obviously— so you cannot judge in terms of people's desire for me now what my life was like before this. But when I think about my past, I've had to conclude that my level of intensity is really male. What lesbians did not like about me was my *intensity*. They really couldn't deal with it, whereas

straight women—because they are used to
dealing with men—never had a problem
with me. It took me years and years and
years before I saw this ... All I know is
that I never connected with lesbians. I
mean, I talk very fast, but even when I
wasn't opening my mouth, there is something about me that just was not interesting to lesbians. Men, on the other hand,
have always been interested in me, but
my problem with men is that I refuse to
play any games of nursing and caretaking
and all the stroking you have to do to keep
men going from day to day. What I want
from men is good sex—virility.

SB: One thing I wonder as I read interviews
with you is whether you've been through
anything similar to what I have been in
my own lesbian sex life. I had sex with
women for years, where I was very inhibited because of what I thought would be
offensive as a feminist. I didn't want to
objectify women. I didn't want to be like
a man. I didn't want to be unequal. All
these things bothered me a lot, and looking back on it, it was just plain old inex-
perience and Catholic uptightness.

CP: I had the opposite problem in that I
was trying to be dirty with women and I
wasn't finding it. I was having a lot of
trouble finding women who wanted just

sex. My entire inability to relate to lesbians appears to be due to the fact that I was looking for sex—and they weren't. In the lesbian world you can't just walk into a bar. Oh no! You have to get into a sort of "musical chairs" group where you have to either play volleyball or do things with them or hang out with them.

SB: Isn't it like that anyplace else, though?

CP: Oh, no. That's certainly not the case with men's bars at all. The people arrive there as strangers looking for sex and it is absolutely admitted that the men are looking for sex—that has always been the case, and I find that so wonderful about men, that they don't even pretend that they are looking for friendship. It is a bold admission of desire.

SB: (Laughter.) Have you ever had what you would consider anonymous sex?

CP: Yes, but mostly with men. I was looking for it with women but I wasn't finding it. *That* is the story of my life—it's hilarious. I think that is my destiny—like the Ancient Mariner—to go through this wasteland and to suffer. . . .

The Paglia-Bright anecdotes are supported in *American Couples,* a 1983 survey of six thousand straight and gay couples by the late Dr. Philip Blumstein and Dr. Pepper

Schwartz. They found that lesbian lovers had far less sex than married or cohabiting women. In fact, forty-seven percent of lesbians living together for ten years or more had sex just once a month or less. In contrast, the figure for married women was fifteen percent and for the cohabitors seven percent. "The low frequency of sex at every stage of lesbians' relationships poses crucial questions about the nature of female sexuality," observed the authors. Actually, what the lesbian finding suggested is that without the goad of hunter-men, women tend to revert to the erotic nest where kisses and cuddles often can substitute for orgasm.

Alone in arguing for women's natural nymphomania was Dr. Mary Jane Sherfey, perhaps the most imaginative theorist in recent orgasmology. Although she took Kinsey's famous marriage course as an undergraduate at Indiana University, she abandoned his zoological approach to human sexuality for the realm of psychiatry. As a young physician, she specialized in the uncharted evolutionary significance of premenstrual tension, a line of inquiry that led her deep into the origins of sex itself.

In 1961 Sherfey began reading about an important though neglected discovery in endocrinology, the so-called inductor theory, which stated that in mammals the male fetus is derived from the female, and not the other way around as biologists had universally supposed. According to tests performed on rabbits in the fifties by French endocrinologist A. Jost, the early embryo is all-female and without the subsequent appearance of male hormones every mammal would be born female. Prior to Jost, it was assumed that the embryo was innately bisexual and that male and female structures developed unequally with the former seeming to dominate the latter, that is, the smaller clitoris was regarded as a rudimentary phallus. It was this old-fashioned view that led Freud to demean clitoral eroticism and champion the vagina.

The inductor theory fairly exploded in Sherfey's brain. "I knew what I had to do," she wrote in her cause célèbre book *The Nature and Evolution of Female Sexuality* (1973). "I had to bring this startling revelation to the attention of psychiatrists in such a way that they could not ignore it. To my mind, this meant that I first had to bring this fact to the attention of the psychoanalysts because the Freudians had always been the chief theorists of psychiatry and because this embryological fact would strike a body blow at the Freudian concepts of female sexual development, one of the few original theories of Freud that have remained unchanged since he wrote about them."

Before Sherfey could confront the Freudians, she had to tackle their sacred idea of vaginal orgasm. And everywhere she looked, she saw problems. For instance, she could not isolate any physical reason for this phenomenon in either monkeys or human females. And it made no sense to her that, as Freudians thought, "only a few superior women have the highly evolved or trained cortex to produce the vaginal orgasm." She recoiled from the notion that "the majority of women remain biologically inferior, retarded in their psychosexual evolution compared to men, not sufficiently involved emotionally and intellectually to achieve the vaginal orgasm."

And then in 1982 she found the smoking gun while browsing through a 1960 copy of The Western Journal of Obstetrics, Gynecology, and Surgery that carried an article on female sexual physiology by a then-unknown team named Masters and Johnson. This was a few years before their work would be published in *Human Sexual Response*. "I knew it was a major breakthrough in the study of human sexuality," she wrote. "Then I ripped through all subsequent journals to see if more articles had appeared. I found the second one, and in the last issue just put on the shelf, the study of the clitoris. It was truly a Eureka experience for me. This was it! Freud was wrong. Men were wrong. Women were wrong.

Common sense was wrong. There was no such thing as the vaginal orgasm as heretofore conceived."

Sherfey, who had quit her teaching post at Cornell Medical School for the freedom of private practice and research, became intoxicated with Masters and Johnson's data on the extremes of female orgasm. She was impressed by their description of test women who had fifty consecutive orgasms with a vibrator and their private communication about a sample of approximately fifty previously nonorgasmic wives who were allegedly turned into multiple-climax people after a few days' treatment in St. Louis. These data remain unpublished.

Combining Masters and Johnson's discovery of an underground orgasmic volcano in women with similar evidence of high sex capacity in female primates, Sherfey advanced a unique theory: "The more orgasms a woman has, the stronger they become; the more orgasms she has, the more she *can* have. To all intents and purposes, *the human female is sexually insatiable in the presence of the highest degrees of sexual satiation*" (emphasis Sherfey's).

Sherfey speculated that women's capacity for repetitive orgasm must have been actualized sometime in prehistory. But how to account for the apparent loss of this legacy? Sherfey guessed that long, long ago civilization-building men were the founding fathers of frigidity. She wrote:

> . . . it is conceivable that the *forceful* suppression of women's inordinate sexual demands was a prerequisite to the dawn of every modern civilization and almost every living culture. Primitive woman's sexual drive was too strong, too susceptible to the fluctuating extremes of an impelling, aggressive erotism to withstand the disciplined requirements of a settled family life—where many living children were necessary to a family's well-being and where paternity had become as important as maternity in maintaining family and property cohesion. For about half the time, women's erotic needs would be insatiably pursued; paternity could never be certain; and with lactation erotism, constant infant care would be out of the question.
>
> There are many indications from the prehistory studies in the Near East that it took perhaps 5,000 years or longer for the subjugation of women to take place. All relevant data from the 12,000–to–8,000 B.C. period indicate that precivilized woman enjoyed full sexual freedom and was often totally incapable of controlling her sexual drive. Therefore, I propose that one of the reasons for the long delay between the earliest development of agriculture (c.12,000 B.C.) and the rise of urban life and the beginning of recorded knowledge (c. 8,000–5,000 B.C.) was the ungovernable cyclic

sexual drive of women. Not until these drives were gradually brought under control by rigidly enforced social codes could family life become the stabilizing and creative crucible from which modern civilized man could emerge.

Sherfey has not won many converts and her untimely death prevented publication of a sequel study. Apparently, most sex researchers and anthropologists regard her hypothesis as too fanciful. Anthropologist Donald Symons pointed out, in his book *The Evolution of Human Sexuality,* that the ethnographic record contains no evidence of sexually insatiable females in today's preliterate tribes, including the free-loving Mangaians.

Still, there is a nagging question. If female orgasm itself is evolutionarily unnecessary and benignly neglected by natural selection, where did women's multiple climax come from? Symons has an explanation: "The ability of females to experience multiple orgasms may be an incidental effect of their inability to ejaculate." Citing Kinsey, he noted that preadolescent boys can have repeated orgasms on the same arousal curve. But these strings of climaxes occur in the absence of ejaculation since the glands of young boys have not matured enough to cause emission. Concluded Symons: "The female [multiple] orgasm may

be homologous with the orgasm of the preadolescent male, which occurs before the capacity
for successive orgasms—among a minority of
individuals—is eliminated by the development of ejaculatory ability."

But what if Sherfey were right? What if nature intended women to be as coitally minded
as men or even more so? Should we look back
to pre-civilization, as Shere Hite and other
feminists insist, for a model of modern sexual
harmony? One doubts the model would work
today. There is something about constant
availability that tends to smother ardor in the
married male for his wife, and to a lesser extent, vice versa.

The curve of marital passion seems to de-
scend steadily with every decade—according
to Kinsey, the average rate of intercourse
drops from three times a week in the twenties
to once a week in the forties. Without tension
of *some* kind, the monster of habit, it would
seem, devours romantic feelings.

Abigail van Buren was hip to the notion of
sexual fatigue in a famous column wherein
she quotes a happy, God-fearing husband:
"When the kids were little, our family doctor
wrote on a prescription pad: 'One weekend,
every six weeks, get a sitter for the kids, buy
a bottle of wine, check into a motel with your
wife and treat her like a hooker. And don't
say you can't afford to. You can't afford not

to.' Today our children are educated, well-adjusted and independent, and I am left with a loving, exciting wife."

The letter was signed—"Christians Should Be Lovers." Abby replied: "Dear Christian: Right on. And so should Jews, Buddhists, Moslems, Hindus, etc."

Rather than fantasize about better intercourse through "cultural transformation" as Hite demanded in *The Hite Report,* perhaps it is wiser to play with the basic formula as Kinsey, Hite herself and Edward Eichel have done.

CHAPTER 2

The Search for Female Coital Orgasm

Prior to the twentieth century the *ars amoris* was no art in the West. While natives on several continents and ocean islands carried on without shame, though not without taboos of their own, the more inhibited people of Europe and North America, controlled by patriarchy, restrained by religion and unenlightened by medicine, were especially deficient lovers.

But before putting the blame on sinister forces for spoiling the joys of sex past, one should remember that the erogenous zone was an unsafe place in history. Without prophylactics or antibiotics, venereal disease spread like the plague. Childbirth itself was a huge killer, and those women who survived were frequently and horribly maimed by primitive obstetrics. And woe to anybody who had a sex problem, because there was nowhere to go for decent advice.

Some of the great male minds of Europe believed that sex was just another form of evacuation, thus the horrific medieval maxim about women being "temples built over a sewer." In the sixteenth century the wise Montaigne observed in his *Essais* that "Venus, after all, is nothing more than the pleasure of discharging our vessels, just as nature renders pleasurable the discharges from other parts." This excretory view endured until the modern era.

With ignorance so vast and the status of women so low, female orgasm was not even, so to speak, on the table. A fraternity of dunces in nineteenth century Europe denied that proper ladies even possessed erotic desires. "I should say that the majority of women (happily for society) are not very much troubled with sexual feeling of any kind," declared British surgeon W. Acton in his influential 1857 volume *Functions and Disorders of the Reproductive Organs*. Moist vaginas, like erect clitorides in the seventeenth century, were attributed to lasciviousness and luxurious living.

Backing up the notion of a second-rate arousal grid was a supposed epidemic of frigidity. Sexual numbness, one of the unflattering terms that male doctors gave to females' lack of desire for intercourse and the absence of pleasure therein, allegedly affected the majority of women. New York City was a reputed hotbed of *anhedonia* (Greek for no fun), another clinical term of the day. According to a 1907 article in The Pacific Medical Journal, three out of four married women in this country's then largest metropolis were frigid, though Jewish wives were said to be rarely so.

Actually, a warring theory, also enunciated by men but cherished as well by the opposite sex, argued that women had a more exalted sexual nature. Ovid (43 B.C.-A.D. 17) introduced this feminist concept in *Metamorphoses*, a collection of mythological tales, in which Zeus and his sister, consort and queen, Hera, debate which gender more enjoys sex.

"You females get more pleasure out of loving than we poor males do," Zeus insisted. Hera thought otherwise. And so they consulted a soothsayer named Tiresias, who agreed with Zeus and was blinded by Hera for saying so.

Bold witness for Tiresias was repeated by many authors from the early Christian fathers, who warned against the sirens of sin, to German physician and reformer Iwan Bloch, who made the acquaintance of women who climaxed from merely gazing at erotic pictures and statues. In *The Sexual Life of Our Time and Its Relations to Modern Civilization* (1908), Bloch wrote that "in most cases the sexual coldness of women is in fact only apparent, either due to the concealment of glowing sexuality beneath the veil of outward reticence prescribed by conventional morality, or superior else to the husband who has not succeeded in arousing erotic sensations which are complicated and with difficulty awakened . . . The sexual sensibility of women is certainly different from that of men, but in strength it is at least as great."

As the twentieth century dawned, the good idea of a flaming female sexuality slowly began to drive out the bad idea that women could never be like men in the alacrity of their response. And every orgasmologist, whether oriented toward Freud or toward the tougher-minded science of sexology, seemed to have a different answer to the question of the perfect fit, which was what women really wanted.

WILHELM REICH:
CRAZY VERSUS SANE ORGASMS

According to an old Irish saying, when sex is good, it's the most beautiful thing in the world, but when sex is bad, it's still pretty good.

Wilhelm Reich was German, not Irish. He believed that good orgasms were the key to health and happiness, but bad orgasms depressed him. Actually, this weird scientist and sex reformer, who died half-mad at the age of sixty in Lewisburg Federal Penitentiary in 1957, invented the colossal idea of climax in excelsis and he blamed much of human misery on the failure to achieve it.

Reich's notion about cosmic sexual climax swept into history with the publication of *Function of the Orgasm* in 1927. He was thirty years old at the time and a member of Freud's inner circle in Vienna. Thinking that he was following the founding father's line on the direct connection between mental and genital problems, Reich dedicated the original manuscript "To my teacher, Professor Sigmund Freud, with deepest veneration," and presented it to him on Freud's seventieth birthday.

Freud was not pleased. Though he praised the book as "rich in observation and thought" in a brief note to his protégé, he poked fun at Reich behind his back. Of course, orgasm was important to Freud. After all, he had written in "Sexuality in the Aetiology of the Neuroses" (1905) that "no neurosis is possible with a normal *vita sexualis*." But he did not overly concern himself with the explosive event. As long as men ejaculated in the right orifice and women had vaginal climax, the subject did not materially interest him.

Nor did Reich's farfetched solution to the mysteries of body and soul. "We have here a

Dr. Reich, a worthy but impetuous young man, passionately devoted to his hobby horse, who now salutes in the genital orgasm the antidote to every neurosis," Freud wrote to a mutual friend, Lou Andreas Salome, in 1928.

Where did Reich get his near-apocalyptic concept of orgasm? As psychoanalysts tend to do, he beheld the universe in his patients when they confirmed his deepest convictions. Reich started pondering orgasm in a serious way after noticing something unexpected in a group of male patients. When he asked them about their masturbation fantasies he assumed that they would recount pleasant images of intercourse. Instead, the men reported sadistic or masochistic fantasies that left them discontented after ejaculation. "In not a single patient was the act of masturbation accompanied by the fantasy of experiencing pleasure in the sexual act," he wrote in "The Specificity of Forms of Masturbation" (1922).

Reich next probed the coital attitudes and sensations of hundreds of male and female patients. What he found apparently convinced him that intercourse would always be a quagmire for neurotics. None of the women had vaginal orgasm; and the most potent men felt something like disgust when they climaxed. Reich concluded that *all* patients suffered from incomplete genital satisfaction.

His argument was a stretch, and he was

forced to admit that not a few patients appeared to have hale and hearty orgasms. Still, he clung to the insight that some orgasms were better than others and, more important, that the quality of release separated the well from the sick. His supposition was reinforced in his private life. After a sexually frustrating period in medical school, marked by melancholy after the act, he fell in love with an Italian woman and, at last, had fulfilling sex.

But Reich needed a theory, something on the plane of the Oedipus complex, to explain his unorthodox, practically Copernican interpretation of orgasm. He felt he discovered it in Orgastic Potency, which he defined in *Function of the Orgasm* (1927) as "the *capacity for the surrender to the flow of biological energy without any inhibition,* the capacity for *complete discharge of all dammed-up sexual excitation* through *involuntary pleasurable contractions of the body.* Not a single neurotic individual possesses orgastic potency; the corollary of this fact is the fact that the vast majority of humans suffer from a character-neurosis." (emphasis Reich's)

The corollary was the problem. It was all right for psychoanalysts to visit afflictions on the wounded in their practice—that was an occupational hazard—but it was another thing to call almost everybody else "orgasmically disturbed." Reich dared to assert that having

second-rate climaxes, a condition labelled "orgastic impotence," was "the most important
characteristic of the average human today,
and—by damming up biological (orgone) energy in the organism—provides the source of
energy for all kinds of biopathic symptoms
and social irrationalism."

This, coupled with radical sexual politics
and a tropism for controversy, led him down
a long path of ridicule, rejection and exile. He
was banished from the psychoanalytic movement, deported from Norway and hounded
into prison by the American Food and Drug
Administration for distributing his notorious
"orgone energy accumulator," a box the size of
a telephone booth that purportedly captured
a "primordial cosmic energy" for the cure of
common colds, cancer and impotence.

Reich was surely no Alex Comfort, but he
gave step-by-step instructions for attaining ultimate orgasms. First, one needed to be "unar-
mored," that is, "muscularly relaxed and
physically unblocked"; but after that it was
just a matter of method. Basically, his advice
was—don't do what neurotics do in bed. They
were fast and frantic, violent and stiff, narcis-
sistic and sad *post coitum*. (Neurotic men were
said to have painful erections and neurotic
women to have watery vaginal secretions.
After sex, they were leaden and exhausted,
and often could not sleep.)

On the other hand, Reich's lovers were warned to be slow and easy, men gentle and women active. In "Orgasm as an Electrophysiological Discharge" (1934), Reich referred to "spontaneous and effortless frictions" that focused excitement on the genitals. There was no fear, no fantasy, no rough talk, only surrender to the other.

As tension mounted in the penis and vagina and orgasm arrived, Reich's heavy-breathing, heart-pounding couple were overwhelmed by involuntary contractions spreading from the genitals over the whole body. Immediately afterward, tension disappeared and a warm, melting sensation emanated from the pelvis to the limbs. "The complete flowing back of the excitation toward the whole body is what constitutes gratification," he concluded in *Function of the Orgasm.* "What continues is a grateful tender attitude toward the partner."

Although Reich did not insist on joint climaxes, he assigned simultaneity top status: "In both sexes, the orgasm is more intense if the peaks of genital excitation coincide. This frequently occurs in individuals who are able to concentrate their tender as well as their sensual feelings on a partner."

Reich supplied no proof that his soft strokes and vanilla intentions were essential for maximum sex. "Orgastic Potency" had no more underlying credibility than Freud's "mature" vaginal orgasm. In fact, Reich's blueprint contradicted two historic maxims of the *ars amoris*: that variety is the spice of sexual pleasure and that resistance is the engine of arousal, especially in and around intercourse.

Speaking for erotologists of every era, Comfort observed in *The Joy of Sex* that "being stuck rigidly with one sex technique usually means anxiety." As for the psychology of excitement, even Freud, who could be something of a fogey, recognized that *tension* was an indispensable aphrodisiac. "An obstacle is required to heighten libido; and when natural resistances to satisfaction have been insufficient men have at all times erected conventional ones so as to be able to enjoy love," he declared in the marvelously titled article, "On the Universal Tendency to Debasement in the Sphere of Love" (1912).

Nevertheless, Reich's theory of Orgastic Potency and his orgasm formula, like many other erotic myths, have refused to die. During the Age of Aquarius they were passed on to the human-potential movement and spread through Esalen-style encounter groups. Apparently no Reichian has ever put his mentor's central theory to the scientific test: "It has to be stressed that there are still no scientific studies, from Reich or anyone else, comparing a large number of orgastically potent persons with orgastically impotent ones," commented Dr. Myron Sharaf, author of the Reich biography, *Fury on Earth* (1983).

Perhaps the difficulty was the size of the orgastically potent pool. As Sharaf acknowledged in *Fury on Earth,* even a true disciple like himself achieved the big Reichian blowout only rarely. "I believe that until his last years," wrote Sharaf, "Reich was overly optimistic about people achieving orgasmic potency through Reichian theory or through more sex-affirming social attitudes."

HAVELOCK ELLIS: LONGER INTERCOURSE IS BETTER

Havelock Ellis (1859–1939), the lapsed British physician who advanced sex research in the English-speaking world with his compulsively readable if much censored seven-volume *Studies in the Psychology of Sex* (1936), was an advocate of women's natural amorous instincts. Conceding a widespread coital tristesse among European wives, Ellis blamed inept husbands who paid little attention to the elaborate network behind female excitement.

"Naturally the more complex mechanism is the more easily disturbed," Ellis remarked in an essay, "The Sexual Impulse in Women," published in his second volume. "It is the difference, roughly speaking, between a lock and a key. This analogy is far from indicating all the difficulties involved. We have to imagine a lock that not only requires a key to fit it, but should only be entered at the right moment, and, under the best conditions, may only become adjusted to the key by considerable use. The fact that the man takes the more active part in coitus has increased these difficulties; the woman is too often taught to believe that the whole function is low and impure, only to be submitted to at her husband's will and for his sake ... The grossest brutality thus may be, and not infrequently is, exercised in all ignorance by an ignorant husband."

Ellis, who was wedded chastely to lesbian feminist Edith Lees for twenty-five years, may never have experienced intercourse. His autobiography, *My Life* (1940), is reticent on that particular, but it is clear that Ellis was a sexual eccentric. Although he avoided writing about penetration or male climax, he devoted one hundred pages of his third volume to undinism, his neologism for the clinical term urophilia—lust for urine. In fact, in his private life he was classicly undine (from the Latin *unda*, wave). His idea of an exciting date was having a pee with a female companion, perhaps accompanied by mutual masturbation. "He could love his sweetheart more thrillingly by contemplating a rose at her side than many a man does through coitus," wrote his last lover, Francois Lafitte, to a disapproving Margaret Sanger.

Nevertheless, in spite of his uneasy ways with romance, he was acutely sensitive to the complaints of women. Although he said inexcusable things such as "their brains are in their womb," he promoted women's sexual liberation in his books. In his essay on the female impulse, contained in *Studies in the Psychology of Sex*, he quoted at length the following letter (July 21, 1947) from an anonymous lady who explained why she and her Victorian sisters remained unthawed so much of the time:

I do think the coldness of women has been greatly exaggerated. Men's theoretically ideal woman (though they don't care so much about it in practice) is passionless, and women are afraid to admit that they have any desire for sexual pleasure.

... Even in the modern novels written by the "new woman" the longing for maternity, always an honorable sentiment, is dragged in to veil the so-called "lower" desire. That some women, at any rate, have very strong passions and that great suffering is entailed by their repression is not, I am sure, sufficiently recognized, even by women themselves.

Besides the "passionless ideal" which checks their sincerity, there are many cases which serve to disguise a woman's feelings to herself and make her seem to herself colder than she really is. Briefly these are:—

1. Unrecognized disease of the reproductive organs, especially after the birth of children. A friend of mine lamented to me her inability to feel pleasure, though she had done so before the birth of her child, then 3 years old. With considerable difficulty I persuaded her to see a doctor, who told her all the reproductive organs were seriously congested; so that for three years she had lived in ignorance and regret for her husband's sake and her own.

2. The dread of recommencing, once having suffered them, all the pains and discomforts of child-bearing.

3. Even when precautions are taken, much bother and anxiety is involved, which has a very dampening effect on excitement.

4. The fact that men will never take any trouble to find out what specially excites a woman. A woman, as a rule, is at some pains to find out the little things which particularly affect the man she loves,—it may be a trick of speech, a rose in her hair, or what not,—and she makes use of her knowledge. But do you know one man who will take the same trouble? (It is difficult to specify, as what pleases one person may not another. I find that the things that affect me personally are the following: [a] Admiration for a man's mental capacity will

translate itself sometimes into direct physical excitement. [b] Scents of white flowers, like tuberose or syringa. [c] The sight of fireflies. [d] The idea of the reality of suspension. [e] Occasionally absolute passivity.)

5. The fact that many women satisfy their husbands when themselves disinclined. This is like eating jam when one does not fancy it, and has a similar effect. It is a great mistake, in my opinion, to do so, except very rarely. A man, though perhaps cross at the time, prefers, I believe, to gratify himself a few times, when the woman also enjoys it, to many times when she does not.

6. The masochistic tendency of women, or their desire for subjection to the man they love. I believe no point in the whole question is more misunderstood than this. Nearly every man imagines that to secure a woman's love and respect he must give her her own way in small things, and compel her obedience in great ones. Every man who desires success with a woman should exactly reverse that theory.

As Ellis saw the sexual predicament, if women were not juveniles, or too long unflowered after first youth, or traumatized by honeymoon hell, they were ever ready to climax, but only in harmonious circumstances with the right, *unhurried* man. In spite of his

learning on the variations of coitus, Ellis coun-
seled no particular position or technique. Instead, men's timing was everything to him.
"In coitus the orgasm tends to occur more
slowly in women than in men," he wrote in
Studies. "It may happen that the whole process of
detumescence is completed in the man before
it has begun in his partner, who is left either
cold or unsatisfied."

Eschewing Freud's mumbo-jumbo about clitoral versus vaginal orgasms, Ellis simply prescribed an increase in male staying power.
"There can be no doubt whatever that very
prolonged intercourse gives the maximum
amount of pleasure and relief to a woman,"
he declared in *Studies*, citing twenty-minutes-
plus matings of Hindu, Moslem and Javanese
men and women, as well as Jews and Negroes,
who were said to be pleasurably slow to ejaculate. "Not only is this [slow is better method]
the very decided opinion of women who have
experienced it, but it is also indicated by the
well-recognized fact that a woman who repeats the sexual act several times in succession often experiences more intense orgasm
and pleasure with each repetition."

TH. H. VAN DE VELDE: MEN GIVE WOMEN ORGASMS

Dr. Th. H. Van de Velde, Ellis's contemporary, likewise preached the tortoise-approach in order to bring inexperienced women to "full erotic efficiency." He felt that intercourse was a matter of good sportsmanship. "When the two participants in the act are so unequally equipped," he attested in *Ideal Marriage* (1926), "the more apt and active must do what the superior in a contest of speed or skill does. He handicaps himself in order to preserve the woman's interest and assure her pleasure in coitus."

The Dutch gynecologist ascribed frigidity to genital infantilism in the women of Western Europe and the United States, a geographic anomaly left unexplained. But he had a remedy—the more intercourse, the more the clitoris would grow. "In this respect," he observed, "practice makes perfect."

But Van de Velde gave women a role as well. Since highly aroused men had their limits, which he did not specify, and since women are more adaptable, which he did not illustrate, he expected them to accelerate their climax through, again, practice.

Van de Velde had a novel hunch about the origin of female orgasm during intercourse. As this excerpt from *Ideal Marriage* indicates, he, ultimately, gave the credit to men:

. . . in normal communion the man's ejaculation gives the signal for the woman's orgasm as well as his own.

But this again may happen in two ways. The final reflex in the woman may receive its signal from her realization of the muscular contractions of the man's orgasm; or from the impact of the vital fluid.

In any case the significance of the second is very great: and the greater, the more tender and fervent the woman's love. It forms a fit and perfect final link in the wonderful chain of love processes. Those who forget or ignore it have an inadequate and distorted view of this phenomenon.

But only women themselves can declare which of the two—orgasm convulsion or ejaculation— is the talisman which heralds their supreme ecstasy.

And here, individual differences become apparent at once. There are women who decisively affirm that they only experience the orgasm if and when they feel the impact of the seminal fluid against the *portio vaginalis*. But they are in an unmistakable minority. And it is possible to prove this, for the fact that— in adequate and satisfactory conditions—the feminine orgasm almost always occurs immediately after the man's ejaculation, even when this cannot be felt as focused on the *portio*, or when the fluid is very slight in amount— shows that the particular type of sensation is not by any means necessary or universal.

Incidentally, as a back-up for those moments when genital friction failed to bring women to climax, the doctor, who was too reserved to discuss the "genital kiss" (cunnilingus and fellatio) in *Ideal Marriage,* recommended manual manipulation, and quoted the figleaf endorsement of an 1870 manual for French confessors: "If the husband should withdraw after ejaculation, before the wife has experienced orgasm, she may lawfully at once continue friction with her own hand, in order to attain relief."

ALFRED KINSEY: STEADY, UNINTERRUPTED RHYTHM

For Kinsey, rampant frigidity was a figment of naïve imagination. Based on a sample of approximately twenty-three hundred married white women in *Sexual Behavior of the Human Female* (1953), he contested Van de Velde's notion of widespread coolness in American beds. Kinsey's average wife climaxed during intercourse about seventy-five percent of the time. Four out of ten did so always or almost always in the first year of marriage. By the twentieth year, that figure reached forty-seven percent. After thirty years, only ten percent appeared completely impervious to the peak.

Fourteen percent of all women in the sample had regular multiple orgasms.

"Our discovery about the rate of coital orgasm didn't get the attention it deserved," Gebhard said recently on the telephone. "People focused more on our statistics about premarital and extramarital sex."

Kinsey remarked that young women got off to a sluggish start compared to young men—ninety-nine percent of the latter were having three orgasms a week while half of the former were still waiting for their *first* one—but their response steadily heated up as they lost inhibitions and gained experience. Cutting through a morass of psychiatric alibis such as penis envy, castration fear, defense against incestuous wishes, aversions to menstruation, coitus, childbearing, etc., Kinsey pointed to harder evidence to explain the wide variation in female response.

Kinsey argued, first of all, that females were built differently from one another. Although all healthy women were potentially orgasmic, some were better at it than others (e.g., those who climaxed regularly, multiply or from little or no stimulation) thanks to, he thought, more finely tuned nervous systems.

Age was another important factor. The older women became, the more coitus led to orgasm, which also suggested that the sexual substrate, a victim of evolutionary slight, could be improved by exercise.

Kinsey also found that premarital orgasms had significant correlation with the marital kind. The more orgasmic a woman was before marriage in either petting, masturbation or coitus, the more orgasmic she was later on. However, Kinsey admitted that it was not possible to prove cause and effect because it was likely that the more responsive women were the ones who were having it all before the wedding anyway.

Gebhard said that the most interesting connection involved coital orgasm and a woman's generation. Women born before 1900 were significantly less orgasmic than their daughters born thirty years later. "It seemed that the older women were more inhibited than the younger ones," he said. "This meant culture was an important influence on female sexuality."

Although Kinsey was short on the how-to, there are a few passages in both reports that bear on technique. In the male volume, Kinsey went against the perceived wisdom of the sex doctors (some of whom called swift ejaculators neurotic or pathological) and applauded the fleet mammalian reactions of American men. Three-fourths of his male subjects were finished within two minutes, while women often needed a quarter of an hour to become fully aroused. For Kinsey, a rapid ejaculator was a symbol of mammalian strength, "however inconvenient and unfortunate his qualities may be from the standpoint of the wife in the relationship."

But Kinsey changed his tune about women in the female volume after analyzing the data on masturbation. To his apparent amazement, women who required twenty minutes of stimulating intercourse to climax were much faster with their own hands. For example, half of the women in his sample who masturbated climaxed within three minutes and many of the rest deliberately lingered to extend the pleasure. Kinsey's male masturbators, on average, took just a few seconds more. This discovery—that women were not appreciably slower than men to climax—convinced Kinsey that sexologists like Ellis and Van de Velde were looking in the wrong place for the answer to female coital orgasm. Frigidity was not a matter of timing after all. "It is true that the average female responds more slowly than the average male in coitus, but this seems to be due to the ineffectiveness of the usual coital technique," Kinsey asserted.

Did he have something better in mind? Regrettably, he was vague on the subject except for one piece of advice given in his volume on female sexuality—steady stimulation without interruptions:

Response in the female, and for that matter in many a male, may not depend on elaborated, varied, and prolonged petting techniques as often as upon brief but uninterrupted pressures and/or continuous rhythmic stimulation which leads directly toward orgasm.

Our data even suggests that the use of extended and varied techniques may, in not a few cases, interfere with the female's attainment of orgasm. Most females are able to masturbate to orgasm in much less time than it takes them to reach orgasm in coitus which is preceded with extended foreplay, because masturbation is usually continuous and uninterrupted in its build-up to orgasm.

... Moreover, because she is less aroused by psychologic stimuli, the female is more easily distracted than the male in the course of her coital relationships. The male may be continuously stimulated by seeing the female, by engaging in erotic conversation with her, by thinking of the sexual techniques he may use, by remembering some previous sexual experience, by planning later contacts with the same female or some other sexual partner, and by any number of other psychologic stimuli which keep him aroused even though he may interrupt his coital contacts. Perhaps two-thirds of the females find little if any arousal in psychologic stimuli. Consequently, when the steady build-up of the female's response is interrupted by the male's cessation of movement, changes of position, conversation, or temporary withdrawal from the genital union, she drops back to or toward a normal physiologic state from which she has to start again when the physical contacts are renewed. It is this, rather than any innate incapacity, which may account for the female's slower responses in coitus.

"The biggest enemy of intercourse is thinking," says Gebhard, who once observed that sixteen minutes of to-and-fro was sufficient to satisfy a woman. "Just when a woman is enjoying a position and building up to orgasm, the man is turning the page thinking about a new position. When you get too fancy, you spoil it. Kinsey favored no particular technique—he thought thrusting was enough."

MASTERS AND JOHNSON:
CLAIMS OF FEMALE ORGASM

Dr. William Masters and Virginia Johnson picked up the torch from Kinsey. The professor from Bloomington had filmed a few people having sex in the privacy of his attic, but the obstetrician and his assistant, an ex-country singer, produced an epic of copulation footage in their St. Louis lab. After going farther than any sexologist had gone before with a camera, they published their data on the physiology of orgasm in *Human Sexual Response*.

For their next project the couple shifted to sex therapy, applying their knowledge of sexual mechanics to the treatment of orgasm-related dysfunctions such as impotence and female anorgasmia—translation, frigidity. Apparently they were extremely adept at solving the sex dilemmas of ordinary "marital units." They claimed an eighty percent success rate for the nearly eight hundred men and women who came to St. Louis for two weeks of intense instruction. When they announced these astounding results in *Human Sexual Inadequacy* in 1970, a new field was born. Masters and Johnson were hailed as miracle workers. Where psychiatry and psychology had failed with their talk-therapy, condemning marriages to sexual confusion and frustration, they prospered with short-term behavioral exercises that trained women and men to climax. Masters and Johnson were so encouraged by their findings that they could write in the preface to their new book: "It is to be hoped that human sexual inadequacy, both the entity and this book, will be rendered obsolete in the next decade."

But stripped of mountains of jargon, Masters and Johnson produced a mouse of a manual. For example, their answer to premature ejaculation was the "squeeze technique" (a woman presses the tip of the erect penis between her thumb and the first two fingers for three or four seconds), which helped men to retard their over-enthusiastic emissions. They acknowledged that the squeeze was a variation of Dr. James Semans's stop-start method already in some vogue.

As for solving "coital anorgasmia" in women, the greatest prize in sex research, they were spare with specific advice. They advocated no special techniques or positions for bringing women to coital climax. Instead, there was a longish description of the two-week treatment program of counseling sessions, non-genital nude massages, light, teasing foreplay, "non-demanding thrusting," considerable "mounting, dismounting and remounting," and shifting from the woman-on-top position to bottom-to-side. How did the eight of ten of their coitally frozen female patients manage to experience orgasm? They did not give a physiological explanation.

The best measure, it is generally agreed, of any therapy lies in its ultimate consequences. "The abiding guide to treatment value must not be how well patients do under authoritative conditions but how well they do under their own cognizance without therapeutic control," Masters and Johnson wrote in *Human Sexual Inadequacy*. "This result finally must place the mark of clinical failure or success upon the total therapeutic venture."

Their initial success rate for anorgasmic women was spectacular; the five-year follow-up figures in *Human Sexual Inadequacy* were even better. But how orgasmic, one wonders, were the success cases? How did Masters and Johnson define success in the real world? Were the women gratified by every intromission or just some of them? We do not have much data. The outcome criteria, the standards by which treatment success and failure are judged and on which Masters and Johnson rested their reputation, were missing from *Human Sexual Inadequacy*. And because other therapists, hewing to their guidelines, were unable to replicate their feats, doubts about the pair's claims tended to simmer during the seventies.

In 1980 two gutsy San Francisco therapists broke ranks in a legend-busting article in the August *Psychology Today* entitled "The Inadequacy of Masters and Johnson." Dr. Bernie Zilbergeld of Oakland and the late Dr. Michael Evans, a collaborator, cited flawed research and reporting, data gaps and the absence of the success-and-failure criteria in *Human Sexual Inadequacy*. They challenged the famed authors but their challenge went unanswered.

Author, sex therapist, and self-appointed

watchdog in an unpoliced occupation, Zilbergeld persisted in his heresy with a critique at the annual meeting of the Society for the Scientific Study of Sex held in San Francisco in November 1982. A young colleague of Masters and Johnson, Dr. Mark Schwartz, approached him and asked why he was acting as though they would not tell him their criteria. Schwartz arranged a meeting the next day for his boss with Zilbergeld, Evans and their friend, Berkeley therapist Bernard Apfelbaum, in a lounge at the Cathedral Hill Hotel.

Zilbergeld asked if he could take notes while Masters and Schwartz disclosed the data. According to Zilbergeld and his witnesses, Masters said that he listed a woman in the success column if she had one orgasm in St. Louis and at least one orgasm during intercourse in the next five years! Zilbergeld says that he read his notes back to Masters, who, allegedly, confirmed their accuracy. "I was so floored," recalled Zilbergeld, "I didn't say anything." If one is to give credence to this exchange, it does tend to diminish the astonishing success rate of Masters and Johnson's program.

In the June, 1973, issue of *Forum* magazine, Zilbergeld recounted his exchange with Masters in San Francisco and criticized the whole field of orgasmology.

Sex therapy, like all therapies, has been vastly oversold. Before going further, let me say that some of the treatments and approaches used by sex therapists today are much more effective—at least more cost-effective—than the methods of the past. But the problem, as I see it, lies in exaggerated claims. For example, I see constant references in the media to tremendous success rates—eighty, ninety, one hundred percent—and that's so misleading.

Sex therapy is especially good with anorgasmic women—that is, women who have not had orgasms—and with premature ejaculation. These dysfunctions submit to fairly simple training exercises. But the results are not so promising with more complex matters like erection difficulties and situational anorgasmia; that is, women who are limited in their ability to climax in different circumstances and positions. Apparently we're not doing well treating desire discrepancies, either.

Incidentally, improvement is not the same as cure—a distinction therapists sometimes forget. The cases they present to the public are always dramatic successes. But, generally, that's not what happens in therapy—sex or otherwise.

. . . All therapists have to drum up business, because there simply are not enough clients for their services. In one way or another we are drawn to those things that give us a chance of making a good living and, if possible, of establishing an empire.

So we find areas where nobody else is working, and often that means we create new myths, new standards and new expectations. As long as people come into our offices with sex-related problems, we assume that we can fix them. That may have been our mistake. The same thing happened with psychoanalysis, Rogerian therapy, behavior therapy.

I think Masters and Johnson will suffer the same fate as the creators of other therapies who have claimed success that was not borne out by later investigation. That's already happened with Masters and Johnson's work. They will be remembered for popularizing brief, symptom-oriented treatment of sexual dysfunctions and for some of their physiological work. But their extraordinary success rate—their statistics on the efficacy of their therapy—is already dismissed as an exaggeration.

These provocative words appeared on the eve of the Sixth World Congress of Sexology in Washington, D.C. (May 22–26, 1983), where Masters and Zilbergeld were bound to collide. Masters' scientific integrity was on the line; he could no longer avoid his Inspector Javert on the matter of the missing outcome criteria.

Standing before a large group of admirers, many of whose careers were based in some degree on the viability of the St. Louis research, Masters denounced Zilbergeld and Nobile (who was then editor of *Forum*), denied having said anything to Zilbergeld in San Francisco about a single-orgasm test for success, and then furnished the criteria and supporting data not included in *Human Sexual Inadequacy*. "The Masters & Johnson Institute has never considered that a nonorgasmic woman who had only one orgasm during the two weeks of therapy in St. Louis and one orgasm during the next five years was a therapeutic success," he said. "The criteria applied to the cases presented in *Human Sexual Inadequacy* were actually that a woman needed to be orgasmic in at least 50 percent of her sexual opportunities to be considered a success."

The ovation was considerable. Though late in coming, the fifty-percent rate was a perfectly valid criterion. The record was now supposedly clear. "A midget can see farther than a giant if he's standing on the shoulders of a giant," commented Kinsey's co-author Wardell Pomeroy in the New York *Times*. "Masters and Johnson are the giants of their field."

In spite of the dismissal of Zilbergeld's criticism, Masters and Johnson were to a degree damaged by the controversy over their statistics. In his address to the Congress of Sexology, Masters did not account for why he did not include his perfectly valid definition of success in *Human Sexual Inadequacy,* a neglect that carried through ten printings. When asked by Nobile to explain, Masters replied that he simply forgot.

It is not just Zilbergeld's word versus Masters' word in San Francisco. Both Dr. Evans and Dr. Apfelbaum (who was trained at St. Louis and presumably had no axe to grind) backed Zilbergeld's version, while Masters' two witnesses, Schwartz and another colleague, refused comment.

Masters and Johnson's last book was *Crisis: Heterosexual Behavior in the Age of AIDS* (1988), co-authored with their colleague Dr. Robert Kolodny. The couple charged that the deadly HIV was "running rampant in the heterosexual community" and could be spread through casual contact. They faulted the AIDS establishment for "benevolent deception" and "misinformation" and advocated the prophylactic of premarital testing.

They received a great deal of criticism. At a post-publication press conference, Masters was unable to defend his assertion that AIDS had broken out of the high-risk groups to the extent claimed. "I simply believe this," he stated on ABC-TV's "Nightline."

The therapeutic work of Masters and Johnson is rather more creed than science. They may well *believe* that women climax from the pulling of the clitoral hood, that they cured eighty percent of their previously frigid female patients, that they changed homosexuals into heterosexuals, and that AIDS can be casually contracted, but they have not faced peer review or engaged in real dialogue with their critics, leaving their most interesting claims unproven. And that is to be regretted, since the couple, who are now divorcing, are no doubt well-meaning and conscientious people.

SHERE HITE:
A NEW KIND OF INTERCOURSE, OR ELSE

Shere Hite made a bestselling impact in 1976 with *The Hite Report: A Nationwide Study of Female Sexuality.* The work contained many quotes on the ways women gratify themselves and the ways men control the erogenous zone. Her scholarly image was diminished from the beginning (*People* magazine commented that her work was to sexology "what sunglasses are to acting,") but she assuredly hit a feminist nerve in the popular culture. Suddenly this former exotic model with an M.A. in history from the University of Florida and two semesters of doctoral courses at Columbia University was mentioned in the same breath with Kinsey and Masters and Johnson.

Perhaps the most controversial sections of *The Hite Report* concern the intercourse-orgasm nexus that bedeviled her predecessors. But Ms. Hite had a surprise twist: "The question

should not be: Why aren't women having orgasms from intercourse? but, rather: *Why have
we insisted that women* should *orgasm from intercourse?*," she declared, upsetting the apple-
cart of sex therapy (emphasis in original).
She excoriated men for an "almost hysterical
fixation on intercourse and orgasm." She ignored Kinsey's insights on the female substrate and downplayed his news about the
average wife's climaxing three out of four
times in coitus because Kinsey counted the
times that orgasm was hand-assisted. By
dwelling on the seventy percent of her much-
questioned sample that reported coitus did
not consistently produce orgasm, she was able
to represent intromission as a patriarchal plot
designed to keep men on top in more ways
than one. (Respondents to the first questionnaire were recruited from readers of *Oui,* the
Village Voice, and from the women's movement, a group that almost all would agree does
not necessarily represent the general female
population.)

According to Hite, Masters and Johnson
were the enemy because they assumed that coital orgasm was desirable for women and they
made it look easy. Hite passed over their alleged success in treating coital anorgasmia
just as she avoided dealing with Kinsey data
that contradicted her agenda. She ridiculed
the description of female orgasm in *Human*

Sexual Response: "Masters and Johnson's theory that the thrusting penis pulls the woman's labia, which in turn pull the clitoral hood, which thereby causes friction on the clitoral glands and thereby causes orgasm sounds more like a Rube Goldberg scheme than a reliable way to orgasm."

She was on firmer ground, however, when she remarked that the methods that excited Masters and Johnson's highly orgasmic test-women could not be projected onto the rest of the female population.

In spite of Hite's disdain for the act, she provided an informative primer to coital orgasm by delineating six clitoris-heavy methods that her respondents—the happy thirty percent—climaxed from copulation. Kinsey had hinted at the basic formula—much steady pressure on the clitoris—but Hite was more specific about technique in *The Hite Report:*

Orgasms during intercourse in this study usually seemed to result from a conscious attempt by the woman to center some kind of clitoral area contact for herself during intercourse, usually involving contact with the male's pubic area. This clitoral stimulation during intercourse could be thought of, then, as basically stimulating yourself while intercourse is in progress. Of course the other person must cooperate. This is essentially the way men get stimulation during intercourse: they rub their penises against our vaginal walls so that the same area they stimulate during masturbation is being stimulated during intercourse. In other words, you have to get the stimulation centered where it feels good.

Hite felt strongly about clitorally correct intercourse. If men did not get it, they should be evicted from bed.

Hite reprised her anti-intercourse theme five years later in the 1981 *Hite Report on Male Sexuality*. According to 7,239 responses, *homo Americanus* felt pretty good about his sex life. "There was hardly a man in the entire study who did not report that his sex life was better than it had ever been before," Hite declared. But she also detected trouble in the bedroom: "There is a gut feeling on the part of most men that something is wrong—that although there are beautiful elements to sex as we know it, somehow there are unnecessary problems, too."

Hite's solution to America's sexual malaise was a return to a prehistoric—that is, matriarchal—state of affairs, in which, she argued, intercourse, especially with the man above, is not the *sine qua non* of the art of love. Although eighty-seven percent of the women in the female *Hite Report* liked intercourse, as did almost all of her male sample (thirty-five percent of whom preferred being on the bottom), Hite knew better. "Intercourse," she insisted, "is a celebration of 'male' patriarchal culture," and therefore must be suspect. Despite the testimony of 7,239 men, *The Hite Report on Male Sexuality* seemed to be about what Shere Hite wants. Although the book's myriad methodological and statistical problems refuted the pretension of serious research, it brilliantly fed the national appetite for sex confessions. The testimonies, culled from a questionnaire of 168 essay questions, were a feast of all-American erotica. Often eloquent, sometimes banal, Hite's respondents discoursed throughout eight long chapters on such topics as male identity, extramarital sex, intercourse, masturbation, men's view of women and sex, rape and pornography, homosexuality, and sex and the older man.

Since men have never been reticent about their prurient interests, the disclosures in this report were less arresting than those in the volume on female sexuality. Consequently, the surprises were few. Yet the shocks of recognition were many. In the first chapter, on growing up, Hite recorded the sins that he-man fathers visit on their sons. One man explained:

"Men are trained at an early age to disregard any and every emotion, and *be strong* [emphasis in original]. You take someone like that and then wonder why they don't and sometimes can't express feelings. Not only that, they are supposed to be a cross between John Wayne, the Chase Manhattan Bank, and Hugh Hefner."

Hite dealt with male-female relations in the second chapter. Astonishingly, seventy-two percent of her married respondents tried extramarital sex after just two years of monogamy. This huge rate is probably the result of biased sampling, but the reasons for infidelity rang true. Most of Hite's adulterers complained of too little sex at home, while others blamed the boredom of too easy access to their wives. Hite figured that these reasons cancel each other out. Refusing to accept the word of wandering husbands, she cited a hidden, unconscious anger toward women as the real cause of extramarital affairs.

The heart of the book was an eight-page brief in the third chapter, titled "Intercourse and the Definition of Sex." Here Hite criticized the patriarchal culture of the West for forcing the otherwise polymorphous desires of males into a mania for intercourse.

Hite did not seek to banish intromission from the amorous art, though she would prefer to have men back off from their single-minded devotion to the act. When she asked the question, "Would you like to change the definition of sex so that it was not so rigidly focused on erection and intercourse?", most of her respondents failed to understand the query. Given this uncomprehending state of patriarchal sex, Hite longed for a matriarchy, where intercourse would not be king.

Hite whipped herself into an anti-patriarchal frenzy over the man-above posture. "During traditional intercourse, the ancient patriarchal symbolism of the man on top comes to the fore: the man on top, 'taking' his pleasure, the whole force of the social structure behind him, telling him what he is doing is Good, Right, and that he is a Strong Male—with the woman looking up into his eyes, not resisting and hopefully [*sic*] celebrating these feelings with him, saying yes, you are great."

While emphasizing the cultural imperatives of intercourse, Hite neglected biology—as if genes had nothing to do with our sexual situation. Donald Symons, author of *The Evolution of Human Sexuality*, cut through Hite's historical explanations: "It's simpler to suppose that men tend to seek and enjoy intercourse for the same reasons that other animals do," Symons told Nobile. "These dispositions evolved over millions of years because they promoted reproductive success. Hite ignores cultural anthropology and thousands of ethnographies showing that intercourse is the *sine qua non* of sex everywhere."

Hite returned in 1987 with *Women and Love: A Cultural Revolution in Progress.* Prefaced by tributes from colleagues and backed by 102 pages of statistical charts, the book was attacked by critics who fastened on her claim that "70 percent of women married more than five years are having sex outside marriage."

Upset, understandably, by bad publicity, Ms. Hite was on the verge of a media breakdown when she slapped a limo driver who called her "dear," walking off a TV show and even pretending to be her own publicist under an assumed name.

JOHN PERRY: HITTING THE G SPOT

Before the ink was dry on Shere Hite's 1981 volume on *Male Sexuality,* a book appeared that brought back the old intercourse with a Freudian vengeance. *The G Spot and Other Recent Discoveries About Human Sexuality* (1982), by Alice Ladas, Beverly Whipple and John Perry argued that women had a hitherto-unrecognized erogenous zone in the vagina that caused deep vaginal orgasm and, in some cases, ejaculation.

Such claims were revolutionary to orthodox orgasmologists who believed that female excitation centered on the clitoris.

Despite the weight of accumulated research from Kinsey, Hite, and Masters and Johnson, John Perry, a psychologist and expert on vaginal muscles, dared to dissent. It takes some nerve to say, as Perry did to Nobile shortly after publication, that he and his coauthors had located an erotic *terra incognita*. "We tend to believe that the area of the G spot includes a vestigial homologue of the male prostate."

Perry felt that most sexologists have ignored the importance of the G spot, an erotically sensitive zone located two inches inside the vagina on the anterior or front wall, first described by Dr. Ernst Gräfenberg in 1944.

Perry, an ordained minister, believes that God put the spot in the vagina to make intercourse more pleasurable for women. He elaborated on his theory in a conversation with Nobile in *Forum* (September, 1982).

"Common folk knew it was there," Perry said. "It is only medical science which has been confused for the past thirty years. In the 1930s and 1940s, the American sexologist Robert L. Dickinson acknowledged patients' reports of both vaginal and clitoral orgasms, but he was unable to find medical explanation for the vaginal kind. Then Kinsey came along and concluded that only the clitoris was sensitive, and Masters and Johnson assumed that Kinsey was right. But we now know that Kinsey's experiments were flawed. They used a Q-Tip to test for sexual responsiveness, and naturally the clitoris responded much more than the vagina did. We discovered that you have to apply deep manual pressure to the wall of the vagina to get a response from the Gräfenberg spot—and that's much more like what happens during intercourse."

When asked to describe the spot in detail, Perry seemed less certain. "The G spot is probably composed of a network of blood vessels, the paraurethral glands and ducts, and nerve endings which surround the urethra near the bladder neck," he continued. "It is a vestigial homologue to the male prostate gland. It is usually found halfway between the back side of the pubic bone and the front edge of the cervix, along the course of the urethra. If there isn't too much fatty tissue, the urethra often feels like a piece of wet macaroni."

Why wasn't Perry sure? "For two good reasons, the necessary research hasn't yet been done. First, the tissue we're talking about is extremely delicate, and most anatomical studies are done on the cadavers of elderly women whose Gräfenberg spot has long since degenerated. If all we knew about the penis was what we could glean from elderly cadavers, we might never suspect what it was like in its erect state.

"Second, the G spot shows considerable variation in size, shape and location. It may be smaller than a dime, or larger than a quarter. But the main reason is that no one has bothered to investigate the questions before now. Most anatomists agree that the tissue is homologous to that of the male, but they never addressed the question of its purpose.

"They [Masters and Johnson] have only questioned whether it ought to be called the 'female prostate.' I think they still believe that all orgasms involve the clitoris, too. A few weeks ago Masters told me he could not understand the source of the tremendous amount of fluid that some women claim to ejaculate upon orgasm.

"During our gynecological examination, one almost always finds an area that fits the description. We haven't found but a few exceptions in several hundred examinations. Many physicians have trouble finding it the first few times, but as they get experienced they get more proficient.

"You see, the standard pelvic exam never uncovered the Gräfenberg spot because the physician passes right by it, looking for pathological conditions. He can ask the woman, 'Is this tender?' 'Is this sore?' 'Does this hurt?' But the doctor is never allowed to inquire if his touch feels good.

"If he said, 'Does this turn you on?' most women would jump off the table and run out the door. And he would be reported to the medical ethics committee. Testing for sexual sensitivity in the vagina is simply not part of a standard gynecological examination. That's the province of sexologists."

Careful not to slip into unethical conduct while searching for the G spot, Perry got his test-women to sign consent forms and arranged for female physicians to do the examination. Sometimes there was spontaneous orgasm: "It [the spot] is usually easiest to locate if you let the woman guide you. She can feel the exceptionally pleasurable sensations before the spot begins to swell. In some women, the swelling is extremely pronounced. If stimulation is continued, some women will have an ejaculatory orgasm even during the exam. There is a letter in our book from a woman who says that even a normal pelvic exam is embarrassing for her, because the speculum presses on her G spot and she always comes when the speculum is opened."

If the G spot exists and if it is so sensitive, why don't women all climax during intercourse? How could such a wondrous thing be shrouded in mystery all these centuries? Perry was on less than firm footing when he tried to explain the history of the spot: "Many more women would have orgasms during intercourse if sexologists hadn't told them that they couldn't. Dr. Helen Singer Kaplan is a good example of that. I think women were clearly destined by the Creator to have orgasms during intercourse. But since sexologists have told them not to expect it, they don't.

"Hite was taken in by Masters and Johnson. 'Masters and Johnson have proved that all orgasms are clitoral,' she wrote in the female *Hite Report*. Now, that statement is misleading. Masters and Johnson never *proved* [emphasis Perry's] any such thing—they just assumed it. And Hite was selective in what data she used."

Why would Hite be biased on the site of orgasms?

"I don't know—maybe a personal preference," he said. "Unfortunately, the clitoris has gotten tied up in sexual politics. Some feminists have mistakenly taken the stance that the clitoris needs to be elevated to a position of equality with the penis. Ironically, that was Kinsey's position, too.

"As a psychologist, I must stress the point that sexual response, just like any other bodily function, is mostly 'learned.' How these different orgasms would be experienced if our heads weren't influenced by the pontifications of sexological theorists, I don't know.

"The G spot orgasm, they say, is deeper inside them and more emotional. We think women have elements of both kinds most of the time. This is very important; most orgasms of most women are 'blended' most of the time.

"Fortunately, most people don't listen to the experts, most people just go ahead and enjoy life. Only the intellectuals get screwed up by what we experts say. Ironically, it is better-educated women who accept the 'clitoral only' theory who have trouble with vaginal orgasm."

Actually, the G spot is a mammalian throwback because it encouraged the animal position.

"The 'best' position is any one in which the woman is in control of movement, because she can direct penile pressure to where it feels best," Perry observed. "Also, the 'doggie position' is often recommended because, as Elaine Morgan noted in *The Descent of Woman*, the reproductive machinery was designed back when we were quadrupeds.

"Most animal intercourse is rear-entry, which happens to be a perfect position for stimulating the G spot. The G spot can be hard to find—that's only because we have a predilection for the missionary position. In rear entry, for example, it is easy to find—it's natural."

Perry stated that the supposed link between the G spot and ejaculation is the major theory of his book:

"The G spot is connected through the pelvic nerve to the spinal cord and back again to the uterus—this pathway accounts for ejaculation.

In the case of males, the experts agree that the pelvic nerve is what triggers the prostate gland. All we are saying is we think females can work the same way as males. More research is needed. But we have a very clear hypothesis—the so-called Skene's glands, or paraurethral glands, the homologues of the male prostate."

Women would ejaculate more regularly, speculated Perry, if nature and their lovers had encouraged their potential: "First, it appears that only the male ejaculate has reproductive significance, so evolution favors males who ejaculate. Second, we have reports from many, many women who say that they have been severely criticized by their male partners for ejaculating, and so they have learned to suppress the response. Our society is very intolerant of natural body secretions and odors. We also believe that there has been a change in female ejaculation over the past century. In 1926 Dr. Van de Velde wrote in *Ideal Marriage* that half the men in the world believe that women ejaculate. Today perhaps 10 percent do. That could reflect a comparable change in what women are actually allowed to do in society.

"Our work has certainly made vaginal intercourse scientifically acceptable again. For thirty years sexologists have been deprecating vaginal orgasm and intercourse. Based on a mistaken reading of Masters and Johnson, science made it seem ridiculous for the female to like intercourse. What I mean is that we have made the desire for vaginal orgasm acceptable to women again; and we have also vindicated those women who are natural ejaculators, who were told that they were just urinating. We have hundreds of letters from women saying, 'Thank God—finally there's a scientific explanation for what I've been ridiculed for all these years.'

"A third thing is that males and females are more alike than different. Many of the differences in the ways women respond sexually— such as taking longer to orgasm—are not the result of anatomy but social training.

"Now that it is acceptable for women to ejaculate, let's see what happens over the next twenty years. Maybe as many women will ejaculate as men—and just as quickly and often, too."

The sex establishment attacked the trio of authors for what they called an unscientific haste to publish in the popular press before submitting to peer review. "I feel outrage at what I perceive as the irresponsible, premature assertion of embryonic findings and creative, but carelessly developed, ideas as facts ..." wrote researcher Jeanne Warner in *The SIECUS Report,* a publication of the Sex Information and Education Council of the United States.

Bernie Zilbergeld joined other critics and wrote in *Psychology Today* (October 1982): "The smell of a bestseller was in the air. A large advance was offered; Perry and Whipple, joined by psychologist Alice Ladas, rushed to get into print, several years before such a move could be scientifically justified. The result is a disaster. *The G Spot* is full of poorly supported claims and half-baked ideas, lacking in thought and care, and certain to cause a lot of needless suffering."

The feminists at the Boston Women's Health Book Collective were wary: "It's a relief for those women who feel a urethral gushing of liquid during orgasm to find an explanation for this apparent 'ejaculation' and for some others to find what may be another source of pleasure," they conceded in the *New Our Bodies, Ourselves*. "However, if a G spot orgasm becomes a new 'ideal' for the sexually liberated woman, or is used to reinstate the so-called 'vaginal' orgasms as superior, it will become a new source of pressure, making us feel inadequate or unaccepting of our own sexual experiences." The best analysis of the G spot controversy can be read in Janice M. Irvine's *Disorders of Desire* (1990).

In 1983 Dr. Teresa Crenshaw, an influential San Diego sex therapist, announced that she had discovered the first clinical evidence of the G spot in the cadavers of ten women between the ages of forty and sixty-five. "While we can't say for sure, because we don't have a large number of studies, I think it's fair to conclude that all women have a prostate gland just like all men do," Crenshaw said in the San Diego *Tribune* (July 26, 1983).

Without waiting for these results to be reported in the literature or replicated by other researchers, the authors of *The G Spot* took Crenshaw's rather premature claim as vindication. "*The G Spot* may be the most important book on human sexuality since Masters and Johnson," they wrote in a letter to the editor in the San Diego *Tribune* (July 26, 1983).

Now, almost a decade later, the G spot has largely faded from the public's consciousness; it still awaits official anatomical recognition quite apart from its reputed orgasmic and ejaculatory powers.

DR. ALAN BRAUER AND DONNA BRAUER: HOUR-LONG ORGASM

While most orgasmologists have concentrated on such basic matters as sexual climax, a married team from Palo Alto pushed matters further in the early eighties with their self-help *ESO*: *How You and Your Lover Can Give*

Each Other Hours of *Extended Sexual Orgasm (1982).

If one is weary of brief climaxes after long, hard foreplay, if one's partner goes to sleep after having his or her orgasm, if one has ever wondered why one cannot climax for a full hour every day of the week while also eliminating headaches and high blood pressure and adding an inch to the penis, Dr. Alan Brauer's prescription is indicated.

After witnessing a primal orgasmic scene of unheard duration, Dr. Brauer, a psychiatrist, went home with his wife Donna, a biofeedback specialist, to duplicate the feat. In consort, they devised techniques of marathon masturbation and called them "extended sexual orgasms or ESO."

For example, ESO for men is one hour of tumescent expectation; for women, it's finger exercises on the G spot and the clitoris. But for the Brauers ESO is an altered sexual state with serendipitous side effects. "Regular ESO—ideally, daily ESO—is the strongest as well as the safest, and certainly the most pleasurable, medicine we know," they stated in the book. "Unlike every other treatment or medication available, ESO is *totally safe*. There are *no* reported bad side effects." (emphasis in original)

They spoke to Nobile about their discovery in their Palo Alto offices just as *ESO,* the book, was being published. Their conversation appeared in the February 1983 *Forum*.

"A couple of our female clients mentioned in passing that they had unusual orgasmic episodes," Dr. Brauer remembered. "Their orgasms seemed to go on and on, and they were very different from their regular orgasms. They described the experience with a sense of awe and puzzlement, which is how it came into psychotherapy. As I recall, the orgasms occurred during intercourse. At the time it wasn't appropriate for me to inquire about details. Then we heard of a couple who claimed that they were experiencing this on a regular basis. And so we arranged to watch them make love. This demonstration of female extended orgasm was extremely impressive.

"There were visible contractions occurring at first, and then they gradually decreased in frequency so that each contraction appeared to last longer. No woman could do that deliberately for an hour. You can try it and you'll see that even if your PC muscles are in very good condition, you're going to quit after about 100 or 150 contractions.

"With this kind of dramatic evidence, Donna and I went home and began practicing ourselves. By trial and error over a period of many months, we recognized that it was possible for each of us to experience ESO. As we got a method down, we started teaching it to clients who came to us with sexual problems and wanted some assistance."

"Every young woman dreams about earth-shattering orgasms," Ms. Brauer said. "And when she finally has an orgasm it is very nice and a release, but it's a boomp, boomp, boomp, and that's it. The earth does not move under her. The waves don't crash on the shore. It's not the magnificent feeling that she was told about."

ESO, on the other hand, was magical and mysterious in new age fashion. Ms. Brauer could not define it exactly, but she surely knew it when she had it: "ESO seems to be like an altered state of consciousness. In a female's mind, it is like floating; no questions, only answers. Your whole body is contracting—not just the genital area—in waves of orgasm, quick sharp waves and longer waves stretching out. It's a state of no resistance. It is a complete letting go."

Although marathon female orgasms are part of the sexology lore, no man has ever ejaculated continuously for minutes, let alone hours. Since male orgasm and ejaculation usually go together except for the very young or the very, very aroused, Dr. Brauer had to change the definition of male orgasm to make it fit under the ESO cap.

"Unlike women, men have a two-stage orgasm," said the psychiatrist. "The first is called the internal emission stage, or the 'point of no return.' That's when the orgasmic reflex is triggered, and about three seconds later it is inevitably followed, so it is thought, by ejaculation, which is the second stage.

"During the emission phase, the prostate, the seminal vesicles and the Cowper's gland are contracting and oozing out the fluids that collect in the urethral bowl. This lasts for a couple of seconds before the muscles at the base of the penis contract, thereby squirting out the ejaculate.

"This process is thought to be totally automatic, and indeed it is. But I operate under the assumption that any reflex that can be measured and sensed can be controlled, which is one of the basic tenets of biofeedback. It occurred to me that the orgasmic reflex—the first experience of emission which is then reflexively followed by ejaculation—might also be controlled. Thus the emission stage occurs without necessarily having the second stage, which is ejaculation. What a man experiences in ESO, then, is an elongated emission phase, but without ejaculation. It is still orgasm, because there are two stages in the orgasmic process."

When asked to comment on the literature that says ejaculatory inevitability is lost at around the age of thirty, Dr. Brauer replied, "The literature is all wrong. The fading sensation of ejaculatory inevitability occurs well be-yond thirty. For most men it's more like the fifties or sixties."

As easy as ESO was supposedly achieved, the couple agreed that not every aspirant is up to the hour-long exercise. "Some people will extend their orgasm from six seconds to maybe three minutes or five minutes or ten minutes, depending on the priority they have on the feelings, the sensations and sex itself," Ms. Brauer said.

Dr. Brauer elaborated: "It depends on how much training you do. We know of people who have orgasms lasting several hours. But we don't set that goal for most people. A more reasonable possibility is something like half an hour, or even less.

"For example, we're pleased if a person is able to prolong orgasm by any amount of time. If they normally have a ten-second orgasm, and after spending some time in ESO training they are able to have one lasting two minutes, we think that's fantastic, and so do they.

"Nearly half the couples achieve what we could define as an extended orgasmic experience. Of the people who come to the seminars, about 15 percent attain what they describe as an ESO experience.

"And we take anything over a minute of orgasm as success; a minute is considered the absolute outer end of normal orgasmic response in current sex therapy literature.

"ESO has probably not been reported because sex researchers considered it impossible. For a long, long time nobody thought a human being could run a mile in less than four minutes. Then there was Roger Bannister. Suddenly a whole slew of people ran faster than four minutes. And now they are talking about running a mile in less than three minutes and thirty seconds."

The Brauers argued that regular ESO practice improves the symptoms of arthritic pain, gastrointestinal complaints, high blood pressure, asthma and skin eruption and alleviates alcoholism, insomnia, drug dependency, explosive anger, as well as adding an inch to the penis.

"If you focus attention on any part of your body, it can get stronger," Ms. Brauer stated.

But longer?

"The penis has the ability to grow because there is a lot of the penis that is buried in the body," she said.

"A number of clients spontaneously reported that they noticed their penises were getting longer," Dr. Brauer added. "I can think of about eight or nine men who reported this. And in at least five of six cases, that was confirmed by their partners. I think that it's a miracle. But it's logical if you think about it."

And what about the other claims?

"ESO itself may not be the sole reason," Dr. Brauer said of the powers attributed to this technique. "It may be going from no sex at all to having orgasms twice a week. Regular orgasms have made a significant difference in the experience of many of these complaints. We find this not uncommonly.

"For example, I saw a woman who had intractable migraine headaches. She was constantly making trips to the emergency room of her hospital for Demerol shots. But when she and her husband began having extended sexual orgasms—it was only a couple of weeks—she had no headaches, nor was she on medication.

"If even 10 percent of our readers find more sexual pleasure than they thought possible, then I feel that we have succeeded."

The doctor's wife agreed with this position: ESO was not everything or the only thing. Nor even the last thing. "If you look at ESO as work, then it is work," she said. "I think of ESO as two human beings who get together for a pleasurable voyage. Learning to have extended pleasure. Learning to have extended orgasm. Learning to care and put more attention on each other, which is what a relationship is all about. And wherever they decide to stop is perfectly fine. There is no orgasmic right or wrong.

"I would hate to think that the pleasure Alan and I are now having is all there is. I would like to always think there's more, because every sexual act we have is different."

This was a pleasant end note to the earlier, rather expansive claims of the couple, as well as their learned predecessors. Indeed there was more to come, as Ms. Brauer hoped, although not in the fashion she expected or through the grandeurs of ESO.

Enter Edward Eichel.

CHAPTER 3

Edward Eichel and the New Intercourse

UNVEILING THE ALIGNMENT

Edward Eichel unreeled a film of his sex technique on May 23, 1983, the first day of the Sixth World Congress of Sexology in Washington, D.C. Eichel was the fourth and final presenter at an afternoon panel session called "New Findings On The Physiology of Sexual Response."

Sitting on-stage with him in Lincoln Room West of the Washington Hilton were Dr. Thomas Lowry, M.D., author of *The Classic Clitoris*, who gave an update on the neurophysiology of the clitoris, and panel chair Beverly Whipple, R.N., co-author of *The G-Spot*, who spoke about "female orgasmic expulsion" (ejaculation). Rounding out the discussion group was Dr. Douglas Mould, a professor from Wichita with a specialty in women's pelvic muscles, who spoke on the role of the "muscle spindle" in facilitating female orgasm.

Eichel's curriculum vitae was the least conventional, least academic of the panelists. His training and background were mostly in the arts, rather than in sciences. He graduated with a B.F.A. from the School of the Art Institute of Chicago in 1958. As a Reichian, he was more visionary than scholarly, more intuitive than deductive, more psychoanalytic than sexological. During the sixties he pursued a career as a painter with some success in Manhattan. But he tuned out the downtown art scene. Temperamentally conservative, even a bit on the prudish side, he was put off by the dionysian. "I saw everything demolished in the Andy Warhol era," he would tell the SSSS board in 1989. "People would masturbate in a store front window and call it a happening."

After turning 40 in the early seventies, he devoted himself full time to psychotherapy. His special interest was compatibility between the sexes and he formulated a theory of "optimal relating" based on something called alignment. In the loose language of humanist psychology, he defined alignment as "a synthesis and balancing of the physical, emotional, and mental factors in relating." He applied his compatibility principles to communication and to sex. For over a decade he developed the alignment, first in encounter groups, then with his marriage therapy clients in Manhattan and later in workshops in several European countries. In 1977, he delivered a paper on his idea at the Third International Congress of Medical Sexology in Rome, crediting his sexual technique with a "synergic effect that rejuvenates the whole psyche." But the slant was too Reichan—Reich was his only citation—to command attention among hard headed sex researchers.

Six years later at the Sixth World Congress in Washington, D.C., Eichel presented a leaner, harder version of the alignment that moved away from his mentor and closer to the realm of sexology. At the time, Eichel had not yet earned his reputation as an iconoclast but he would get off to a rousing start by criticizing Masters and Johnson's research in his presentation. Masters and Johnson had criticized the "coital override" position, the foundation of Eichel's technique, in *Human Sexual Response*. Although Masters himself was in the audience, Eichel felt confident and comfortable when he rose to refute the Great Couple of modern sexology. Whipple, then a supporter of Eichel, made the introduction.

With only fifteen minutes at his disposal,

Eichel got right to his case, which unfolded with the aid of slides and a ninety-second black-and-white film of a couple doing the alignment.

"The documentation that I'm about to present is the result of several years of work with couples in a psychotherapy practice in which each couple underwent a two-year program," he said. "This consisted of weekly psychotherapy sessions, and every third week a sex seminar in which they discussed and formulated what I am calling a *sexual alignment* (emphasis Eichel's). The sexual alignment consists of a positioning that is specifically aligned to give genital contact, a coordinated form of sexual movement—very specifically coordinated—and what I would term *complete genital contact* (emphasis Eichel's), with the inference that there is a genital 'circuitry.' The film that you are about to see was done in privacy. The couple had a remote-control unit and they set the camera in motion themselves." Unfortunately, the equipment misfired, the film did not roll. Eichel then shifted to his slides, which depicted close-up drawings of the genitals during the alignment.

The first slide showed the man riding high on the woman with his penis bent in a north-south direction inside the vagina. This was the initial stage of the alignment, which, remarked Eichel, "differs from what might be

142

considered the normal female supine position inasmuch as the male is up forward. And the base of the male penis—the external base—presses into the clitoris. And direct contact is kept with the clitoris.

"Here we have an enlargement [slide] showing the penis in a normal positioning, where it would not connect to the—it might intermittently or not at all connect to—the clitoris."

Linking the alignment to the late, great sexologist and anatomical illustrator Dr. Robert L. Dickinson, Eichel flashed a drawing of the clitoris in excursion or movement taken from Dickinson's *Atlas of Human Sex Anatomy* (1949).

"This is another diagrammatic presentation where instead of the penis operating upward and downward in the vaginal barrel without contact with the clitoris, here it is up forward rocking on the clitoris. The phenomenon might be called 'clitoral excursion,' as documented by Dickinson. This sketch [drawing by Dickinson] was done in 1929. And, you'll notice here, he has the traction process with the clitoris moving upward and moving downward. Probably in alternate strokes of movement."

Although Eichel devised the alignment before the G spot emerged as an issue in intercourse, he granted homage to the G spot tissue in his discussion.

"This [slide] is a representation more close to the actual anatomy. And there are two particular target areas of stimulation in sexual alignment. One is clitoral contact. And the second has to do with what I believe is the 'G'—the Gräfenberg—spot stimulation.[1] Here you have the clitoris caught in the traction between the female pubic symphysis and the male pubic symphysis, and it would move up and downward as long as the man and woman move in exactly the same degree upward and downward. Both have to supply exactly equal motion. And it has to be coordinated consciously and intentionally.

"It requires considerable discipline to learn this motion," Eichel continued. "The clitoris would then, thereby, move upward and downward. And, initially, I thought that was the only factor that was creating a *synchrony* (emphasis Eichel's). Now synchrony could come even from the fact that the woman's equal movement stimulated her the way we have always known the male's movement stimulates the male. So there was much greater syn-

[1] Contradicting Eichel, anthropologist Lionel Tiger wrote that the man-behind position was better suited to G spot stimulation in *The Pursuit of Pleasure* (1992): "If, as some researchers suspect, there is in fact such a location as the 'G-spot'—a point where the vaginal canal is particularly sensitive, so that vaginal orgasm is more readily experienced—then rear entry will maximize strong pressure on this region from the penis and enhance pleasure all around." Perry, co-author of *The G-Spot*, likewise favored this position.

chrony. When I learned about the interior wall of the vagina, what's termed the Gräfenberg Spot, it occurred to me that *above* (emphasis Eichel's) the clitoris—what is happening— there is a rotation between the male and female monses. And that rotation applies a deep pressure. There is probably even a buckling effect from the cartilage of the pubic symphysis."[2]

Returning to a slide showing the man and woman in the alignment, he added some practical tips for the position:

"One important thing that I might mention is that the male does not hold his weight on his elbows. The whole positioning matters. His weight must be evenly distributed. It must be higher up. And, any tension in the shoulders—let's say from the upper back region—would probably cut off the motility to the genitals. And that would be felt as a cutoff of sensation."

Finally the projector was repaired and the

---

[2]Eichel comments: More recently, I have expanded my theory of G-Spot stimulation to include the woman's urethra directly. In alignment her urethra receives deep and steady pressure. The entire urethra—from the external glans to the internal G-Spot—was identified as a sex organ by Josephine Lowndes Sevely, who published her findings from a Harvard-approved study in 1987. In *Eve's Secrets*, Sevely reports, "The woman's [urethral] glans is not a 'fixed' organ. . . . During coitus, the glans is pressed between the woman's pubic bone and her partner's penis" and "penile thrusting makes the glans slide in and out of the vagina—creating a pleasurable sensation for the woman."

film was ready to go. Eichel commented as the couple in full man-on-top alignment proceeded to climax with only small, slow and smooth pelvic movements. Here he aimed a polite shot at Masters and Johnson for their treatment of the coital override:

"What I might mention is that Masters and Johnson believed that clitoral contact was *impossible* (emphasis Eichel's). And that may be because the male tends to speed up and it's a very taut positioning of the male and female genitalia. So that could be very painful and cause 'rectal and vaginal discomfort.' Also, the pliability of the male penis is much greater than the plastic electric-powered phallus [used by Masters and Johnson] and would be capable of subtle and deep pressure stimulation of areas that would affect the pelvic nerve and the Gräfenberg Spot."

Eichel could not finish his presentation with a dramatic flourish. There were no hard data indicating that his variant of the pelvic override was something special. All he had were the feel-good anecdotes of his clients attesting to extra-intense and often simultaneous orgasms, and his ardent conviction, based on many personal episodes of alignment, that his technique was a milestone in orgasmology. In his heart he felt that he had found the cosmic climax predicted by Reich and had thereby solved the ancient riddle of female frigidity. But without some scientific backup, the alignment was in sexology limbo. Thus, sounding like the ghost of Reich, he completed his brief talk with reference to an unidentified "energy" that purportedly triggered orgasm in aligning couples. "And this [the technique] has almost a bioelectric charge mechanism," he said, reminiscent of Reich's definition of orgasm as an "electrophysiological discharge." "So there's no speeding up or rushing toward orgasm, which suggests the build-up of a kind of a particular increment of sexual energy," he closed.

Without the customary fanfare of statistical claims, the alignment was seen at the time as a position that everybody had attempted at least once in the override mode, but one that had managed to go uncelebrated in history, although Hite was certainly in the area in *The Hite Report.* Word of his unusual film spread through the Congress, but the headlines belonged to the Masters and Zilbergeld confrontation. Actually, Masters walked out on Eichel's talk, perhaps to prepare for his encounter with the Zola of the profession. Obviously, he felt he had bigger things to worry about than having underestimated the override.

Eichel spent the next five years toiling on the alignment. At the suggestion of his advisor at New York University, he sent questionnaires to fifty-eight members of his old encounter group to ask them about the incidence, frequency, intensity and simultaneity of orgasm under the influence of the alignment. Forty-three of Eichel's disciples replied. He then matched them with a control group of couples untrained in the technique. When both groups were compared, Eichel's conviction was borne out.

For example, seventy-seven percent of Eichel's females said that, if they tried, they climaxed with the man-on-top almost always or often compared to twenty-seven percent of the controls. Before learning the alignment only 4.5 percent of Eichel's females always or almost always came in the supine position but this figure leapt to fifty percent afterward. The alignment also intensified orgasm "very much" in seventy-one percent of Eichel's males and 45.5 percent of the females. Furthermore, it increased the desire for sex "very much" in one of three men and four of ten women. As for simultaneity, none of the females reliably climaxed with their partner in man-above coitus before instruction from Eichel, but one in three did so later on.

Were Eichel's data valid? Were the positive effects of the alignment unexplained by chance? There was, indeed, a significant correlation between the alignment and coital, simultaneous and complete orgasms in Eichel's females.

Nevertheless Eichel's thirteen-page article, "The Technique of Coital Alignment and Its Relation to Female Orgasmic Response and Simultaneous Orgasm," did not set the field ablaze when it appeared in the Journal of Sex and Marital Therapy in the summer of 1988. Partly, the reason was that orgasm formulas tended to be considered sexological dinosaurs. If Masters and Johnson could not come up with a sure-fire technique after filming hundreds of wired-up copulations, who was going to believe a neo-Reichian therapist with forty-three patients and one two-minute home movie? Also at work here was sexual politics. Eichel had accused homosexuals on a "Donahue" program of strangling sex research and had alienated himself from a number of his colleagues. Whipple, for example, gave him the cold shoulder after his "Donahue" comment.

A rare moralist amidst a sea of relativists, Eichel hewed to the Judaeo-Christian sexual code and resented the anything-goes attitude of the latter-day Kinseyans who controlled many of the power centers of sex research. In 1987, he had accused Kinsey-oriented gay sexologists of "promoting a 'pansexual agenda' " that "has no foundation in science and is destructive to the health and well-being of the general public." He pressed his complaint against Kinsey and the gays in a talk titled "Heterophobia: A Campaign Against Heterosexuality" at the 1987 spring meeting of the American Association of Sex Educators, Counselors and Therapists in New York.

Shortly after his paper was printed in JSMT, Patrick Buchanan mentioned Eichel in his syndicated column, saying that the psychotherapist was preparing an exposé of Kinsey. A strict Irish Catholic, Buchanan had always disliked Kinsey for preparing the way for the "sex revolution" and was, not surprisingly, only too happy to give an alleged debunker some precious ink.

Since Nobile had often written about Kinsey, and attacked Buchanan's snarling homophobia on "Crossfire", he telephoned Eichel at his apartment on the lower west side of Manhattan and inquired about his book. Eichel argued that Kinsey was not a deity. He said that Kinsey had biased his statistics in an effort to "denormalize heterosexuality" and he pointed his finger at an on-going conspiracy of Kinsey's followers that purportedly blocked research such as his own because it emphasized compatibility between men and women. Two years later, Eichel elaborated on the so-called "Kinsey agenda" in *Kinsey, Sex and Fraud,* which was co-authored with anti-pornography activist Dr. Judith Reisman and Buchanan

colleague, Dr. Gordon Muir. Nobile reviewed
the book in *The Village Voice* and joined Dr.
Tripp in debating Eichel and Reisman on
"Donahue." Though critical of Eichel's politics, he read the alignment paper and realized
that Eichel had attempted a Reichian leap forward in orgasmology. Having wrestled with
Masters and Johnson and Shere Hite, Nobile
decided to look at Eichel's answer to the
$64,000 question of the erogenous zone.

THE ORIGINS AND ASCENT
OF THE COITAL ALIGNMENT TECHNIQUE

It was not an overnight sensation, says
Eichel. The technique evolved instead in his
first marriage in the late sixties. His then wife
was also an encounter-group leader. According
to the open therapeutic manner of the human-
potential movement, the first aligning couple
shared their insights about pleasure with others on the scene.

Eichel is reserved about revealing the personal motives behind his alignment theory,
but like Reich he was concerned with the
need to impose peace on the war between the
sexes.

"I was reading Reich and Freud and finding
resonance in their ideas about the link between the emotions and orgasm," Eichel re-

called. "I was always disturbed by theories suggesting that sex was more exciting when it was impersonal, that numbers were more important than quality. It was my intuition that the problem of sexual compatibility has been largely ignored by most therapies."

Initially Eichel had no high hopes for his technique. It did seem to bring him closer to his wife and he hoped that it could accelerate therapy. "The atmosphere in the group was thrilling," he said. "All of us were undergoing powerful changes. We worshipped honesty and natural highs. We had the special camaraderie of soldiers in battle." But the group drifted apart at the end of the 60's, and in 1971 Eichel's marriage broke up.

Eichel went on to establish his own practice for couples and gradually introduced the technique to his new clients. The results were the same. The alignment unleashed strong sexual and emotional reactions and Eichel initiated a monthly group seminar to discuss the impact on relationships.

"By 1973 I felt sure that I had something concrete," he said. "I started travelling around to see if I could interest other therapists in my research. I met with other 'bodywork' therapists, with neo-Reichians and even flew out to California to meet the sex-therapy team of William Hartman and Marilyn Fithian. They took me out to supper and then suggested that we go back to their place to observe a couple trying the alignment under my direction. Sex demonstrations were part of their repertoire in treating inorgasmia. The idea was to show patients how easy it was. I told them that their couple might fail. The alignment was an emotional event, too, and they shouldn't presume that their model couple could do it easily. But Hartman and Fithian were so cordial that I agreed.

"The three of us watched the couple attempt the technique. The male got into the position and almost froze. 'I don't know what's wrong, but I can't feel anything,' he said.

" 'How can you say you're not feeling anything, you have an excitation rash all over your body,' replied Hartman. But the male did not have an orgasm.

"I don't know what happened. Certainly not everybody does it right the first time. But I was at least sure that Reich was accurate about a correlation between emotions and orgasm, although the theory is much too tight. Some of the most emotionally involved couples in my practice had difficulty with the technique, too. So I stopped thinking about an absolute correlation."

Eichel married Joanne De Simone, a New York educator, in 1976 and moved to London, where they joined the humanistic psychology movement. Along with De Simone, who supported his alignment research and was the second author of the JMST article, he gave presentations on the position in Denmark, Holland, Belgium, and France as well as throughout Great Britain. As it happened, a few of his closest colleagues fell under the influence of Baghwan Shree Rajneesh, the Indian guru. The Eichels decided to come back to New York.

"One day Joanne said to me," Eichel remembered, " 'we've run all over the world because of your research and we have a school within walking distance from our home that gives maybe the only degree in human sexuality in the country.' In the early eighties we both enrolled in NYU's Human Sexuality Program. Our goal was to establish ourselves professionally and give the alignment further credibility with the academics.

"Early on, NYU was a good environment for me. I liked Ron Moglia, my master's program director. I had some questions, hesitations about the field work—like visiting gay bars and such as that—but I felt that I could focus on my own research for my masters project. I didn't agree with everything, but I didn't feel that I had to.

"I went to two of the program's summer seminars abroad. The one in Sri Lanka in 1982 was a delight, but Amsterdam in 1983 was a nightmare. Dereyk Calderwood, the director of NYU's doctoral program as well as a direct intellectual descendant of Kinsey, asked me before the trip to Holland whether there was anything that I found objectionable in the spectrum of sexuality. I said pedophilia. Yet that was the theme of the seminar in Amsterdam. We had guest speakers from the Dutch pedophile movement and adult-child sex was portrayed in a positive light! I disagreed with much of the presentations and became, I suppose, a nuisance in the classroom. Calderwood said to me: 'You're not going to destroy everything that I've built.' I thought that maybe he was just referring to my performance in the classroom. But if I may be somewhat grandiose for a moment, perhaps he really meant the alignment. Calderwood was a card-carrying member of the Kinsey agenda who seemed to treat bisexuality as the wave of the future. I felt I was supposed to be a convert and drop the alignment. As long as heterosexual intercourse was regarded as nebulous and a generally unsatisfying experience by the Kinseyans, which was Calderwood's opinion, my research into coital and simultaneous orgasm went against the grain."

Indeed it did. Actually, Kinsey was sympathetic to the vicissitudes of marital coitus, which, he said in the female volume, did "considerable damage to the effectiveness of the relationship." He called intercourse between husband and wife "one of the most completely mutual activities in which two individuals may engage." He even extolled simultaneous orgasm "as the maximum achievement which is possible in a sexual relationship." In fact, Kinsey wrote a comprehensive 54-page chapter on the topic of marital coitus in the female volume. By showing that females were not appreciably slower in their sexual response and correcting the standard love manuals on the right male techniques for intercourse (i.e., eschewing elaborate moves for "brief but uninterrupted pressures and/or continuous rhythmic stimulation"), Kinsey was a champion of female coital orgasm.

Apart from Eichel's quarrel with gays and his unprecedented assault on Kinsey, the difficulties between Eichel and his critics were philosophical and methodological. Eichel came to the erogenous zone from Freud and Reich and humanistic psychology, in which feelings were supreme. Sexology, on the other hand, presumed to be scientific. Each camp had its blind spots and fringe enthusiasms, making clashes inevitable. In spite of his paper in the Journal of Sex and Marital Therapy, edited by Helen Kaplan, a psychoanalyst, Eichel would have no more luck with the Kinseyans than Kinsey would have had in the Vienna Circle.

Acknowledging his predicament as an outsider and worrying about the reception to his forthcoming paper, Eichel reached out to Dr. Masters in July 1988. The orgasmologist from St. Louis was under criticism at the time. His AIDS book had recently been attacked in the press and his reputation was affected. Even the heretofore supportive Society for the Scientific Study of Sex had ripped off his and his wife's halos in a blistering *j'accuse*. Eichel sensed that he and the beleaguered Masters now shared many of the same adversaries and so he telephoned Masters to express solidarity and seek his advice. Since he had criticized Masters at the World Congress five years earlier and was repeating his criticism in the impending paper, he was, not unreasonably, unsure of his reception.

Nonetheless, Masters was cordial on the telephone. He seemed to appreciate Eichel's condolences regarding the SSSS statement. "Well, I can't do anything about it," he said, defending his AIDS book. "Every time we make a major report to health-care professionals we have to take a beating."

Eichel reminded Masters that they had met briefly in 1983 at the Sixth World Congress of Sexology when he gave a presentation of his technique. Masters said that he remembered. Since that time, Eichel continued, he had completed further research and found that his alignment technique showed significant gains in the attainment of coital orgasm for women when compared to an untrained control group.

"It's very close to the position you called the 'pelvic override,'" he said to Masters, explaining that he had overcome the problems of discomfort and partial engulfment of the vagina by substituting a rocking movement for the usual male thrusting that threw the override off. "This article will be out very soon and it contradicts your findings on that particular issue," Eichel said forthrightly.

"Good, I'll be glad to read it," said Masters.

Eichel was relieved by Masters' attitude and got down to immediate business—sexual politics.

"I had continuous difficulty from the militant feminism/gay groups in terms of my research because it makes intercourse important again," Eichel said.

"Well, all I can say on that score is that if you present anything that's a variation on the theme, you're going to encounter opposition," Masters replied. "You have to expect that."

"Do you feel that I should just ride this out?"

"Well, nothing really can be done anyway," Masters commented wearily. "You just have to take your beating when you disagree with the powers that be."

"Do you recall that somebody stood up at a conference two years ago in St. Louis and told you that you hadn't said anything relevant to homosexuals?" asked Eichel.

"No, I don't really."

"Well, I got up right after that person—and said that I had been in an NYU sexuality program where we were told that we were all bisexual and that we were homophobic if we wouldn't have homosexual relations," Eichel remarked. "And then I said, 'I'm just sort of glad to see somebody who's still interested in heterosexuality.' Well, I broke up the tension. But the fact is that I have seen many meetings disrupted."

"I know, that happens all the time."

"I think my findings are important," Eichel continued. "And, I don't like the attack on you. They're questioning your *entire* research going back to your earliest work and saying, 'Were you ever valid?' And I'm concerned that when my research comes out—"

"They'll do the same thing to you."

"But unfortunately I've criticized your research," Eichel said.

"That's all right," Masters replied. "Don't worry about it."

"If there's anything that I can do conjointly with you in relation to my research, I'd like to turn this around," Eichel said.

Nothing apparently came of the Eichel-Masters connection, but Eichel went public with his anti-establishment protest after the

SSSS rejected his proposal to speak about the alignment at its thirty-second annual meeting in Toronto in November 1989. He flew to Canada to confront the board of the organization and gave an earful to Bill Dunphy, a Toronto *Sun* columnist. "Sitting in the hotel's lobby bar, nursing a 7-Up, Eichel looks like neither rebel nor fanatic," wrote Dunphy. "In his tweed jacket and conservative tie, Eichel looks more like some genial history professor than some obsessive sexual scientist.

"What he is, though," Dunphy related, "is an artist turned psychotherapist who claims to have developed a sexual technique that offers heterosexual partners simultaneous orgasms and greater personal fulfillment.

"And he further claims that his research results are, in essence, being repressed by a vast conspiracy of homosexuals, lesbians and feminists who have co-opted the field of sexology."

What did these groups have against him, Dunphy inquired. Eichel told Dunphy that it was politically incorrect to argue, as he, Eichel, did, that sex was designed for men and women and that man belongs on top. Old-fashioned marital intercourse was supposedly passé with the sexology establishment.

True or not, the SSSS board ruled that Eichel could not speak on the alignment at future meetings because he had done so in the past and the rules required new data, not repeats of previously presented material.

It is now four years after the publication of "The Technique of Coital Alignment and Its Relation to Female Orgasmic Response and Simultaneous Orgasm," and Eichel is still an odd sexologist out. Nevertheless, the CAT itself, apart from the ideology in which it is embedded, is in harmony with the sharpest intercourse insights of Kinsey, Masters and Johnson and Hite. Whether Eichel has discovered the long sought pathway to orgasm, if there is an orgasm heaven, or a "sauce and pickle" variant of intercourse will be decided, ultimately, by ordinary men and women in the privacy of their bedrooms.

AN ILLUSTRATED GUIDE TO THE COITAL ALIGNMENT TECHNIQUE (CAT)

The illustrations in this guide approximate anatomy, positioning, and movement. The "X ray" views of the genitals show positioning. Arrows and broken lines indicate direction and pattern of movement.

Positioning

Partners begin the CAT by assuming the usual missionary position, in which the man is on the supine woman with his pelvis low on hers (see illustration 1). His upper torso is propped on his elbows, holding his weight up off her chest. To avoid fumbling and unnecessary tension getting started, it is helpful if the woman inserts the man's penis in her vagina. In this position the penis in the vagina is at an angle below and out of touch with the clitoris.

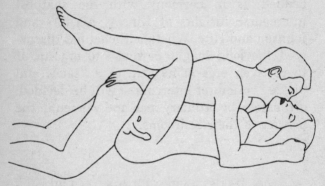

1. The Standard Missionary Position

Next, partners make a small but significant adjustment to get into position for the CAT technique (see illustration 2). The man slides forward higher up on the woman. He assumes the "riding high" posture with his pelvis overriding hers. The base of his penis is brought into direct contact with her clitoris. Taking the weight off his elbows, he lowers his chest, resting his torso on the woman. His head and shoulders veer over her left or right side to a position that is comfortable for both partners. The weight of the man's body gravitates forward over the woman; he should not allow his body to slide backward, causing his pelvis to slip back down under hers. The woman wraps her legs around the man's thighs with her ankles resting on his calves. Her knees should not be raised because that immobilizes her pelvis.

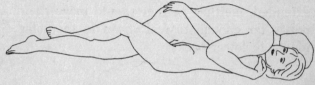

2. The Position of Coital Alignment

Coordinated Sexual Movement: The Upward and Downward Stroke

A rhythm of movement is established in the CAT technique that is interdependent and unique. The motion of one partner corresponds to the motion of the other. The pattern of movement is basically identical for the man and the woman. The upward and downward strokes of movement should travel a distance of about two inches. Movement should not be too hard or too fast. The partners maintain full bodily contact.

The woman leads in the upward stroke of sexual movement. As she exerts genital pressure moving upward (see illustration 3), he offers enough resistance for her to feel clearly defined genital contact with him, but without much force. His pelvis moves only a small distance (note broken line in illustration 3). He does not move backward without her, nor does he move any faster than he is being pushed. His movement is in measured response to his partner's. Her movement upward is not over-extended. Neither partner should move their pelvis far enough to feel strain in the solar plexus or lower back.

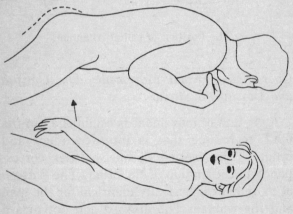

3. The Upward Stroke

The pattern of movement for the man and woman reverses in the downward stroke. The man exerts forward and downward genital pressure (see illustration 4) on the woman's pelvis. He applies only enough force to lead the stroke. The woman exerts moderate but firm resistance, allowing her pelvis to move backward (see dotted line in illustration 4) until it is in a straight line with her spine. The partner moving forward and the partner moving backward exert pressure and counter-pressure. The anatomic design of the male and female genitals and the interplay of the two pelvises allow for the movement to be coordinated in a natural rhythm.

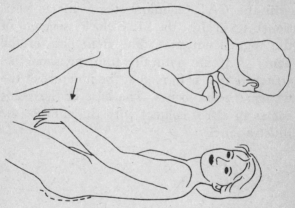

4. The Downward Stroke

Complete Genital Contact

The male and female sex organs together form a genital "circuitry" that is complete when the penis is in the vagina *and* in contact with the clitoris at the same time. Simultaneous pressure and counterpressure during intercourse is critical to keep the penis and clitoris together, and to create a vibrating sensation that helps the man and woman to stay aroused. This contact is established by the positioning and coordinated movement that characterize the CAT technique.

The pattern of movement and stimulation must be held constant throughout the entire buildup and release of the orgasm.

In the CAT technique the penis is positioned up against the "12 o'clock" segment of the vaginal entrance. The front base of the penis shaft fits naturally into the spool-like structure that is formed at the juncture of the woman's pubic bones. The base of the penis comes in direct contact with the clitoris (see illustration 5).

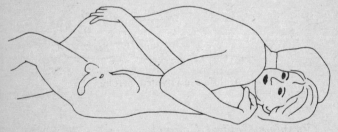

5. Genital Contact in Coital Alignment

There is evidence that the spot at the base of the penis that makes contact with the clitoris is an erogenous zone for the male. It is from this point that the man directs his sexual movement. It constitutes a kind of genital "eye"—an antenna of sensation. For the woman the clitoris is the focal point for directing sexual movement. In combination, the clitoris and the base of the penis act as the fulcrum of the orgasm. Contact between them is maintained throughout the sex act.

The Pattern of Sexual Movement

The Downward Stroke: The pattern of movement in usual coital thrusting is reversed in the CAT technique. In the missionary position the penis slides deep into the vagina when the man moves downward; there is percussion at the end of the stroke when the man can't go any deeper. The pattern of movement is (1) slide, (2) hit. In the CAT technique the pattern of movement reverses to (1) focus, (2) slide. There is a sharp focus of genital sensation as the man reverses the direction of movement by initiating the downward stroke. The woman's pelvis moves downward, and her vagina slides low, leaving the penis shallow in the vagina at the end of the stroke (see illustration 6). This is because the man is positioned high on the woman. Note that the clitoris is pushed upward in the downward stroke of sexual movement.

167

THE PERFECT FIT

Hood of Clitoris

Clitoris

Glans of Clitoris

Labia majora

Urethra

Labia minora

Vagina

Anus

Penis

Vagina

Clitoris

6. Downward Stroke

The Upward Stroke: There is a sharp focus of genital sensation as the woman reverses the direction of movement by initiating the upward stroke (see illustration below). Again, in the CAT technique, the pattern is (1) focus, (2) slide. Her vagina engulfs the penis shaft most deeply as it rises upward. The woman's movement provides for the deepest vaginal "penetration," as opposed to the man moving deeper into the woman, as occurs in normal coital thrusting. Note that the clitoris is pulled downward in the upward stroke of sexual movement.

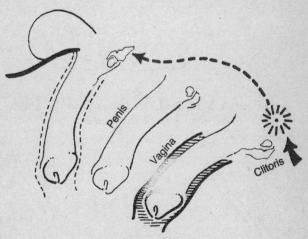

7. Upward Stroke

Principles of Body Movement

The CAT technique depends on fluid movement of the pelvis and spine without additional leverage from pushing, pulling or bracing with the legs or arms. Keep in mind that the spine cannot move freely when there is tension in the limbs and that physical activity cannot be focused in the upper and lower parts of the body at the same time. A transition is necessary from the caressing of foreplay to the coordination of sexual movement. Activity with hands and arms prohibits the concentration of energy in the genitals that is essential in coitus.

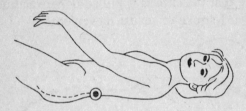

8a. Free Pelvic Movement Originates from the Spine, Without Use of the Limbs.

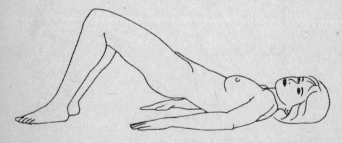

8b. Any Attempt at Leverage by Pulling with Arms or Pushing with Legs Stiffens the Spine and Cuts Off Pelvic Movement.

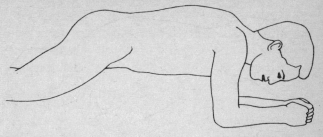

8b. The Man Should Not Support the Weight of His Torso on His Elbows as He Must Keep His Shoulders Relaxed to Be Able to Move His Pelvis Freely.

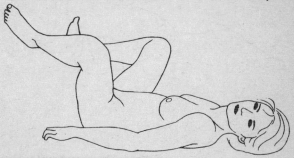

8b. The Woman Must Be Careful Not to Raise Her Knees So High That It Becomes Impossible to Move Her Pelvis.

Partners sometimes have difficulty coordinating the CAT technique—especially in the initial stages of learning the technique—and the man may lose his erection. If so, the couple can adjust their bodies slightly and engage in a few strokes of quicker frictional thrusting until the man is fully erect again. Then they can shift back and resume the CAT technique.

171

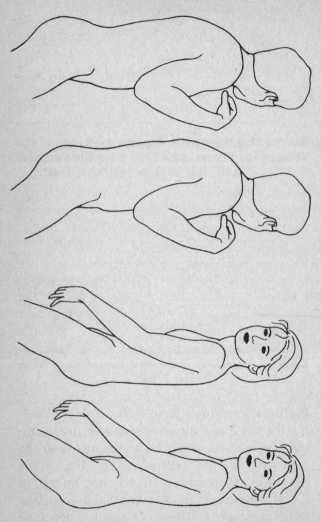

9. Movement of the Spine in Coital Alignment

The Spine in Sexual Movement

The above series of illustrations shows the alignment of the spine and range and pattern of pelvic movement in the CAT technique. Note that the spine is straight and elongated in movement. In contrast, the drawings on the following page show more typical sexual postures and patterns of movement with bending of the spine that limits pelvic movement and interferes with normal breathing. Any erratic or overextended movement that restricts breathing or breaks clitoral contact can result in a loss of genital sensation.

Breathing

To balance the focus and relaxation necessary in the CAT technique, it is important to keep a normal breathing pattern. It is almost reflexive to hold your breath with the build-up of excitement during intercourse. But holding your breath can cut off orgasm or speed it up prematurely. Allow the release of natural sounds during intercourse. Holding back sounds can cause irregularities in breathing. The exaggeration of sounds can also be problematic. It can disassociate one from one's partner. Breathing—like every other part of the CAT technique—requires a delicate balance, which is why the technique requires patience, practice, and a cooperative, constant partner.

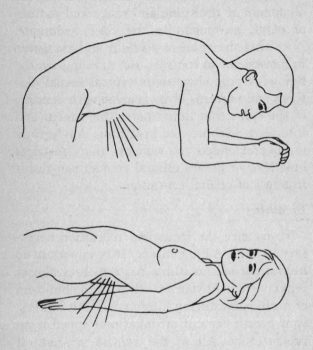

10. Stress in Non-Alignment Postures

Orgasm

The early build-up phase of orgasm requires the conscious coordination of movement. As the couple nears orgasm, the change to involuntary movement begins. The transition from normal control to "letting go" requires relaxation and vulnerability. Partners must try to avoid the archetypal—almost reflexive—tendency to speed up and "grasp" at orgasm, or to slow down and tense up. If bodies are properly aligned and movement is well coordinated, the transition to reflexive movements in orgasm will happen naturally without any disruption.

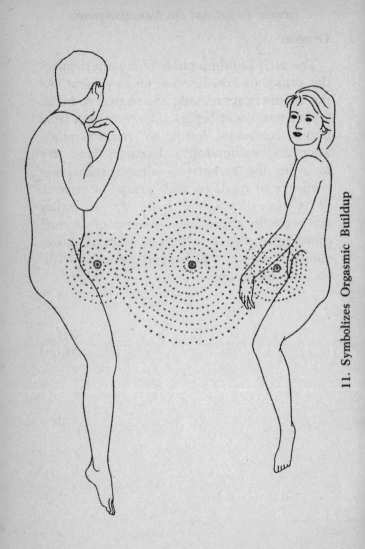

11. Symbolizes Orgasmic Buildup

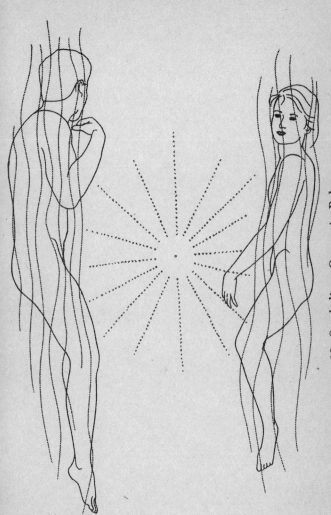

12. Symbolizes Orgasmic Release

CHAPTER 4

Questions and Answers About the Alignment

Q. *Is the alignment easy to learn?*
A. Some get it right on the first try, others take longer. But even if success is immediate, it may not be repeated every time. Coordination is crucial. If the movement is not smoothly done, the man may lose his erection.

Questions and Answers About the Alignment

It's like learning a musical instrument: you may have some luck at first and then you go a bit flat. After that you get more consistency. As a person becomes adept at the technique, it becomes increasingly reflexive and the movement seems to have a life of its own.

Q. *Is adjustment to the alignment more difficult for men or for women?*

A. The position requires coital role reversal for both sexes. Is it harder for a man to give up the instinct to thrust his way through intercourse, or for a woman to be more assertive? Is it easier for a man to soften his movement or for a woman to strengthen hers? A man tends to speed up as he reaches climax, while a woman may not be accustomed to being mobile throughout the act.

The simple and obvious answer is—it depends. But when the alignment goes awry, it is usually because the man reverts to traditional thrusting, and/or the woman breaks the rhythm by slowing down or stopping.

Q. *Why would a man want to give up thrusting in intercourse when it's fun and always leads to orgasm?*

A. Surely, coital thrusting is tremendously enjoyable to men. But some feel that in the process they are doing all the "work." In contrast, with the alignment, the woman controls half the motion, which relaxes the man and increases his range of sensation. The biggest obstacle to the alignment is men who are invested in dominating intercourse and women in submitting. Breaking this archetypal pattern is one of the biggest challenges in learning the alignment.

I distinguish between lust and passion. With lust very often the excitement comes from fantasy. But something entirely different happens with the alignment. There is a kind of calm, a certain tenderness for the partner, partly because you are coordinating with somebody. The *feelings* are just as intense as those associated with more vigorous styles of lovemaking.

Q. *On average, how long does intercourse last with the alignment?*

A. The alignment gives couples a choice. If they want to reach orgasm quickly, say in two minutes, they can. Or if they wish to extend the alignment for ten or more minutes, they can do that, too. A significant number of women said that they had gained control over their orgasm, which allows for both long and short experiences.

Q. *Does a difference in the height of the partners affect the facility with the alignment?*

A. A great disparity in height certainly would not make the technique easier. But the man's body would still be stretched evenly across the woman's. I think a couple could work out a satisfying adjustment just as they do in other positions.

Q. *Does the alignment work with the woman on top?*

A. Yes, but I think the technique is more efficient with the male on top. It is preferable anatomically. According to Masters and Johnson, the clitoris contracts and moves under the clitoral hood prior to orgasm. If the man is on top with his weight leaning on the woman, he is less likely to break contact when the clitoris retreats.

When the woman is on top, this pressure is diminished. From my own experience, it never feels quite as good that way. However, I should say that many people insist that the pleasure is the same no matter who is above or below.

Q. *What about a side-to-side position?*

A. It would be almost impossible for the involuntary part of orgasm—the forward and backward undulating motion—to occur if the bodies are not near-perfectly aligned. That cannot happen when the man and woman are side-to-side.

Q. *What if a man has difficulty achieving orgasm with the alignment, but is happy to bring his partner to climax in the position? Does the technique work halfway?*

A. Sometimes that is what happens. One woman told me that she was totally dependent on the alignment. But after her divorce she fell in love with a man who did not like the position for himself. Yet he satisfied her by using the technique and then reverted to traditional thrusting for his own release. The woman was not delighted, but considered it a reasonable compromise.

I personally think the excitement of the alignment arises from both partners experiencing the same thing at the same time.

Q. *What is so special about orgasm in the alignment?*

A. Every orgasm, of course, is special. But like Wilhelm Reich, I think that some are better than others, and that there are ways to increase their frequency. Reich blamed orgasm difficulties on general sexual repression and said that man had "lost the ability to surrender." It seems to me that the alignment does precisely that—brings about surrender to a new form of lovemaking.

My model, which is indistinguishable from Reich's in many ways, leads to complete orgasm of a certain pleasurable type—that is, the blended orgasm, which combines sharp penile/clitoral sensations as well as soft, melting feelings in both men and women. This is nothing new, I admit. Van de Velde described the combined climax as a mingling of two fine wines. It combines two distinct types of sensation. The first is basically concentrated in the clitoris and the penis and is tactile, sharp, and pulsating as in most forms of masturbation, and like what a man normally feels in intercourse. The second type is a deep, melting pelvic sensation that spreads through the body and is basically the same in women and men.

It may sound strange to hear talk of "melting orgasm" in males. It is much different from the release with ordinary intercourse. Because of the genital stimulation a man receives from the alignment, he can recognize that melting feeling even before he climaxes. Curiously, the literature on male masturbation in the last twenty years has emphasized slower stroking and allowing a more subtle range of sensations, so this idea is not unique to intercourse.

The beauty of the alignment is that it tends to make these *blended* orgasms a much more regular event.

Q. *How is orgasm more "intense" in the alignment?*

A. It is stronger and lasts longer. The climax that comes from quick thrusting can be intense, too, but it is short-lived: it peaks suddenly and then drops off. But in the coital alignment, orgasm builds very slowly. There is no radical climb but rather a sequence of rises and falls—building and tapering in intensity. The peak of orgasm seems infinite. Although it probably lasts only seconds, it *feels* as though time slows down and becomes endless.

Interestingly, when my clients were asked about whether the intensity of orgasm had increased with the alignment, both sexes felt a marked lift, but the men especially so.

Q. *What about simultaneous orgasm? Is that the secret goal of the alignment?*

A. It is more a natural byproduct than a goal. Whenever a woman climaxes during intercourse, the chances of having simultaneous orgasm are very high. But it would be a mistake for couples to try to strive for them. If a couple is making love in the alignment and if their breathing is regular and the movement is coordinated, it is probably going to happen. However, I prefer the term synchronous orgasm because more than timing is involved. There is equal motion and precise stimulation.

It seems the male orgasm has some triggering effect on the female. Van de Velde

so said, as did many of my female clients.
And quite often the orgasms overlap. What
is interesting to me is that when couples
climax simultaneously their body movements seem to harmonize naturally, as if
they were bringing together two halves of
one reflex. When the bodies are perfectly
aligned, which is unlikely to happen *every*
time, the choreography of motion is extremely smooth and maximum stimulation
is continuous throughout the orgasm. The
rhythm leading up to the peak has a regular beat to it. If one person makes an erratic move and the rhythm is broken and
the ensuing release is not synchronous, orgasm may feel like a letdown.

Q. *How can coital orgasm in a woman who may
not usually climax in this fashion be a letdown? Isn't regular coital orgasm the main
benefit of the alignment?*

A. I don't judge the position merely by the
simultaneous standard. Of course, wom-
en's regularity in coital orgasm, which is
bound to increase sexual compatibility, is
the most important contribution of the
alignment. Intensity, synchronicity, monogamous passion, all elements that excited my clients, are perhaps frosting on
the cake and may not be achieved by everyone. The philosophy and the psychol-

ogy behind the alignment is quite distinct from the sexology—it goes *beyond* the physical. My background is encounter-therapy, and so my enthusiasm for the psychic side-effects that I have seen in my practice will, I trust, be forgiven.

Even if the position is a bit "fancy" when performed according to manual detail, just the attempt to learn it can be a revelation. The alignment is an escape from stereotypic intercourse. It is in line with universal opinion from Freud to Kinsey to Hite that steady pressure on the clitoris is a crucial key to orgasm. And, if my experience and those of my clients can be trusted, and I believe they can, the position opens up a whole range of sensations. For example, some of the women told me that they became more orgasmic while learning the technique. It did not matter what they did in bed—masturbation, oral sex, different positions, whatever—after the alignment *all* their climaxes were easier. Apparently, the subtle sensitivity unique to the alignment is transferred to other modes of stimulation.

Experimentation is, I submit, good. The quest for coital orgasm has many mansions. The alignment, which, I realize, will not be to everybody's taste, is one of them— the best one in my opinion.

Q. Yet you recommend using the alignment every time one makes love? Isn't that a prescription for boredom?

A. There is plenty of variety in foreplay. It would be a mistake to think that the alignment prevents pleasuring before the act itself. All of life is, in a sense, foreplay for intercourse. But in my opinion the intensity of orgasm in the alignment is too pleasurable ever to grow tired of it.

Modern sex therapists advise people to do whatever pleases them in bed. We have widened our range of sexual experience and allegedly broken down inhibitions. But we have not resolved the most basic problems of male-female compatibility in sexual intercourse. In spite of our supposed "liberated" sexuality, sex therapists are reporting more and more cases of *inhibited* sexual desire, even a loss of sexual interest in relationships. There is also an even greater advocacy of monogamy in this era of chronic and lethal sexually transmitted diseases. I do, therefore, think that many people at this point in time will welcome new and specific information that can help them to achieve sexual fulfillment in a *committed* relationship.

Q. *Depending on whether you believe Hite or Kinsey, thirty to seventy percent of couples al-*

ready have regular orgasms during intercourse. How then can you call the alignment "optimal"?

A. I believe that there is a design to the genitals that is connected to the design of the whole body as well as to the patterns of motion that the body is capable of performing, particularly the reflexive motions. I am suggesting that there may be a *natural,* that is, an *optimal,* form to the sex act. If the coital alignment is consistently satisfactory for a high percentage of people, this premise should be considered.

Of course, the libido transcends the physical. Easily orgasmic people can attain climax in many different ways. But I am emphasizing reliability for the millions of women who are frustrated by the absence of coital orgasm. Mutuality is also a crucial element: many people who have no trouble reaching orgasm do not connect with their partners.

Q. *At the end of your Journal of Sex and Marital Therapy article you hinted that the alignment could help keep fidelity in marriages in the age of AIDS. Isn't that a large leap?*

A. I should put my cards on the table. I believe that monogamous passion is the healthiest state of sex. I am a Freudian in the sense that I am utterly at odds with the stance that all orgasms are equal and the fashionable defeatist view of some sex therapists and ultrafeminists that heterosexual intercourse is overrated or even dead. No erotic technique can guarantee monogamy, just as no social paradise can promise political harmony. However, I believe that *anything* that enhances sexual compatibility will decrease the sexual tensions that lead to extramarital sex. Since I did not test my sample for that factor, I cannot give you statistics, but the histories of my sample indicate a monogamous desire.

At the very least, the alignment permits a committed couple the opportunity to find complete sexual satisfaction by turning their orgasmic expectations, if they have not already been met, into physical reality. Hite and her sisters cannot say of the alignment what they have said about the old intercourse—that a man is merely masturbating inside a woman if she does not have an orgasm during the act. Dworkin has compared coitus to rape, but the sexes are *equal* in the alignment.

CHAPTER 5

Eight Stories of Alignment and Override

Like intercourse itself, the coital alignment technique is a variable maneuver. Six of the histories recounted here, not including Constance's letter, come from taped conversations with members of Edward Eichel's New York encounter group. They learned the movement and then agreed to fill out a questionnaire on its effects. Eichel used this information for his master's thesis and the article published in the Journal of Sex and Marital Therapy.

Two additional accounts (Miles and Dr. Arthur Schor) show that lovers can spontaneously fall into the alignment or a facsimile with felicitous results.

Eichel's invention is regarded near-reverently by its beneficiaries. Jeff and Jessica asserted that the technique has remade their sex lives, turning intercourse into a long, soothing rush of synchronous ecstasy. Sanford compared his orgasms to a "mellow smile." Ruth called the posture "powerfully egalitarian." Dr. Arthur Schor, a New York psychotherapist who spoke under his real name (all the rest have been changed) claimed that the alignment leads to "timelessness and mindlessness."

These rhapsodies arose from a variety of white, college-educated men and women with a devotion to monogamy and self-improvement. They were primed for success by Eichel himself. So Eichel would not claim that everyone who experiments with the alignment can expect the results attained by his trainees. But the anecdotes supplied by the two people *outside* the therapy group suggest that one need not altogether embrace the theory to take advantage of the CAT position or its variations. Whether a couple is fully or partially aligned, the orgasmic payoff, especially, it seems, for women, can be high.

JEFF AND JESSICA
"The Best Sexual Experience"

  JESSICA: In the beginning, I was in control and had my life together. I was a strong person, and Jeff was the one who needed advice. The situation changed when he started travelling.

JEFF: Our sexual relationship was like a game. Either I was in control or out of control. It was definitely a one-way street. Either I made a sacrifice in bed or she did.

JESSICA: For the first five years we lived out all our fantasies together. When Jeff came back from the road we would be very intense, even flagrant about sex, always trying to keep each other happy.

JEFF: Unfortunately, we couldn't imagine that both of us could have what we wanted without one of us dropping out.

JESSICA: Two years ago I had an IUD removed and we had to find a new form of contraception. I was curious about birth control and had myself charted according to a book on cosmic fertility and rhythm just to find out when it was best to have sex. Neither of us wanted children at the time. When it wasn't safe, we would be turned off.

JEFF: But when it was safe, we would be very turned on.

JESSICA: So intercourse had a lot to do with Jeff's control of himself. Sometimes we would use withdrawal. I was having pretty good orgasms, too.

JEFF: We were having a great time, but in some ways we were working real hard at it.

JESSICA: I remember Jeff was out of town for a month and a friend of mine lent me a vibrator. The orgasms were great, probably just like men's, not the typical flowing back feeling of a woman's climax but sort of flowing forward. I guess it's the huge amount of direct stimulation to the clitoris. So, strangely enough, before coming into the group and trying alignment, although it was by myself and with a vibrator, I had had that sharp male orgasm. It was fantastic, but nothing can touch the alignment now. We had to try it maybe four times. The fourth time we succeeded. It's the best sexual experience ever.

JEFF: We've had simultaneous orgasms previously. It was extremely enjoyable. We'd come together and then Jessica would go her way and feel great and I would go mine and feel great. But when we did the alignment, somehow we never faded away.

The feeling that kept the pleasure going was total genital contact. I didn't even think about the missing friction. I was interested in experimenting with something new.

JESSICA: But there was a kind of friction on the upward stroke.

JEFF: On the sides of my penis?

JESSICA: No, I felt it all around.

JEFF: But the friction for me was all along the top, which was a lot more satisfying. I really got into it right away.

JESSICA: I didn't feel that it was just the contact on the upper side of your penis. For me it was *around* you, and it felt like milking. I can't think of any missing element in the alignment. We tried to get the movement down to a bare minimum, slight, tender and concentrated.

JEFF: Obviously the alignment was a change for us. It was just a lot more sensitive and less straining than any position we had tried.

JESSICA: It was almost as if something kept pulling me in. I would start to feel this frantic thing, I was just out of control. It was very nice but it was intense.

JEFF: I felt this steady kind of contact. It felt nice in the same way, you know, the way a good conversation feels nice. A real good feeling passed back and forth. I tried to stay on top of that without letting the contact dissolve. It was then that I started feeling pleasure. In other words, it took me a while before it started *really* feeling good.

When Jessica came, I was really shocked. But I kept on going. I kept on doing the movement but I couldn't believe it. And I was thinking, where am I right now? Right before I began to come I felt being sucked in like Jessica.

JESSICA: Did you ever ride one of those wooden swings with two seats? One person sits on one side and the other opposite? And you push and then you relax. When the movement is right, I can't think of a better description than that swinging sensation.

JEFF: And neither of us wanted to stop. That's really important.

JESSICA: And even though I was feeling sucked into it, it was like I still had a responsibility to it, as opposed to the vibrator.

JEFF: Even though I was having a lot of pleasure I stayed in control all the time, which is an important part of the contact to me.

JESSICA: Instead of giving into my own sort of frenzy I went with the flow.

JEFF: And I kept a balance with Jessica in the movement without losing any contact, mental or physical. Even at the point of orgasm I was still in control.

Interviewer (Another member of Eichel's group): Control isn't exactly what you mean, I don't think. You are keeping the contact there but letting things happen in your experience. As the orgasm build-up takes place different things happen to different people. For example, as you get close to an orgasm, most people fall off, start giving in to their excitement and climax even faster. They really push it right out, as opposed to continuing to do the thing that you mentioned, which is maintaining a certain amount of focus and letting whatever is going to happen, happen. And not being afraid, not knowing how far it's going to go but just letting it consume you.

JEFF: We were more committed to keeping contact than just getting off.

JESSICA: Afterward I realized that if there had been a fire in the house at the time I could never have escaped. It was precious.

JEFF: Afterward we had this tremendous feeling of sharing that we had never felt before.

JESSICA: We had been looking for something like this for a while because we knew there was something wrong with the old traditional intercourse.

JEFF: No, not traditional. There was something wrong with our ability to go out of ourselves and share with each other. It has to do with sharing.

JESSICA: In a lot of ways the alignment was incredible and amazing, but it was just right for us.

JEFF: Neither of us wanted to continue with the slave model—one of us getting off at a time. I had never even thought of it consciously but I know as I sit here right now I feel a lot better than when we were involved that other way.

REBECCA
A Woman on Top

Sexually speaking, the alignment had an interesting effect on me. Since my divorce from Roger I have taken a leading role in sex with other men. I make love only in the alignment now. I can't get satisfaction any other way. Unfortunately, these men can't understand the philosophy behind the alignment, although they follow my instructions and the physical part is very successful.

I left Roger for two reasons. I was getting in touch with my own being, understanding who I wanted to be and realizing that I couldn't be that person with him. And it had nothing to do with him. But the other reason did—he was unfaithful. For me, monogamy is the most important thing in a marriage.

I'm married now to Tony, who is the antithesis of Roger. The romance is going great and I have really blossomed.

Breathing makes a big difference in the alignment. I notice that if I keep breathing, inhaling and exhaling, that it makes the whole orgasm that much more fulfilling. Teaching my husband how to breathe and tilt his pelvis increased his pleasure, too.

Very few of the women I know, and I know nice women, have orgasms during sexual intercourse. They don't even *recognize* the problem, which I find very strange and depressing. When I tried to tell them about why I learned the alignment, they didn't want to hear about another woman's great sexual experiences. The person that I talked to the most about this is my daughter Elaine. She is one of the two women on this earth that I dearly love. I really want her to appreciate the alignment. She is sexually active. It's important to me that she sees what's possible, that sex isn't just an erotic experience.

Orgasms are all different. Simultaneous orgasm is more exciting and powerful. I've had a dozen incredible orgasms, though I'm not a hundred percent sure whether they were simultaneous. I know the other person had one, but I don't know if it was exactly at the same time as mine. With the alignment, though, you can be sure. You can *feel* it.

I try to encourage doing the alignment more than once in an evening. The second time you're much more relaxed and you've gotten all that tension out and you go deeper.

Tony told me that making love to me is a completely different experience compared to other women. There is a lot of warmth and tenderness and strength that we share during and after sex in the position.

Sometimes I like to be on top. Tony and I are similar in size, so I don't find it uncomfortable. We can still be aligned that way. It's just a reversal of roles. He's an unusual man, very *un*macho. He isn't threatened at all about being on the bottom. I don't know exactly how to describe it, but we're still very aligned with me on top. Other than the fact that he is facing upward instead of downward, if he is moving in the way the female would move on the bottom and the female is moving the way the male would move on the top, it's not all that different. It's not a political issue, merely a matter of doing it differently. But most of the time we do it the other way.

The alignment is not quick and easy. But I'm ever so grateful for knowing the technique. I can assert myself sexually and share it with my husband, even though he didn't go through the process with me. It's not something that I possess alone.

SANFORD
"Simultaneous Orgasm Is Saying I Love You"

It takes two. One person can't do the alignment when the other person is not even *aware*. You can't have one person banging away and the other trying to lock into the alignment. It just isn't going to happen.

As each person feels their strength in the sex act with each other, giving becomes freer. You're not a prisoner of technique, one person feeling they've got to *have*, and the other they've got to *do*. There has to be a sense of *us*. Both have to get theirs and give something in return.

When you're doing it, though, you really can't lose yourself in the other person, you've got to go for your own, too. So in that respect simultaneous orgasm can't be an *obsession*. If you're overly concerned with simultaneous orgasm, you're too worried about the other person. We've had to get away from it and then come back with more perspective. It's been quite a trip going through the group process where that was a sole focus.

I *don't* think the alignment is right for singles—one-night stands and so forth. It's better for couples who *care* for each other but feel there's something missing. It's learning to stir your own energy up in a pleasurable way, at the same time realizing that you're giving pleasure to someone else.

Simultaneous orgasm is, of course, much more fulfilling. I always feel more satisfied if we both come at the same time. Otherwise, I feel something is missing. It's been tough balancing the two—on the one hand wanting mine, getting mine, on the other hand, staying connected and feeling like you want the other person to have hers, too. You go too far in either direction and you can lose it.

Yet one reinforces the other. You get a real spasm going back and forth in waves. It's very nice. My involuntary spasms would actually transfer right to my wife Christine and then cause her to do the same thing. That goes back and forth—involuntarily spasming, just pushing each other's button.

If there's a connection, it surely enhances the act. Otherwise, an orgasm is an orgasm is an orgasm in the masturbatory sense. This connection does not happen every time. It takes a certain emotional and energy level. I can feel when we've got it. I'm sure Christine can, too. It clicks in, you can feel the click in terms of energy. Physically there's a certain connectedness. And, of course, the movement really keeps you in touch with that. It isn't static. It's dynamic.

Christine had her first simultaneous orgasm on the technique. I think she was surprised and happy. Just working at the movement resulted in simultaneous orgasm. We took coming together in the alignment and simultaneous orgasm as one and the same thing.

Simultaneous orgasm for us is kind of a smile. A mellow smile. It's not as serious as the heavy-duty, fast-friction sex that occurs with, to carry on the metaphor, a very severe look. That's the difference between groping with sex and being relaxed on the alignment.

I can't say whether the physical sensation is different. For us orgasm is much more connected to the emotions. It feels like a tickling of all the senses rather than just the penis and lower parts. The emotional aspect becomes part of the physical, so maybe orgasm *is* different on the alignment. And that's where the smile comes in. It's a more *complete* experience, but may be not as earth-shattering because it lacks the violence that other types of sex are supposed to have.

Having orgasm together isn't coincidental. It's more orchestrated. I've noticed that my wife can climax just by sensing that I'm about to, and vice versa. There definitely is a trigger mechanism . . . when you're doing a slow movement, it takes so little to unleash the orgasm, it's like a ballet at that point, if you'll forgive my mixed metaphors. You are so tuned into everything that it's very easy to start it together. I don't know where that triggering comes from. Sometimes I want the movement to go on for hours. Maybe the shared feeling that this is something quite wonderful triggers it. But it would be virtually impossible to have simultaneous orgasm without being aware of the other person's sense and feelings.

For example, many years ago I dated a French woman who used to speak in French during sex. At the time I didn't understand the language. She would announce when she was about to come. I was pretty young and thought that she meant right away, instantly, and I would respond by letting go of myself, and she would say, not yet. She taught me that normally a woman's orgasm is a lot more elaborate than a man's. As soon as she gave me warning, I was able to climax right away, but for her it meant another four or five minutes. I'm afraid I was a lousy lover to her.

Who should try the alignment? I'm a convert, I admit, but certainly people who don't agree that variety for variety's sake is the spice of life and have been frustrated and even intimidated by that philosophy. I think couples who are in love but have sexual problems should surely try it. It's a great message for men who think that women like it only this way or that way. I am projecting my past experience, but I don't think I'm so different or special.

I wonder about the other methods of sex therapy. I know a lot of people who find they're deeper and deeper in their problems rather than cured. I don't suppose, though, that the alignment cures all problems either. It's minimally an early education on how to treat the opposite sex. If a sixteen-year-old boy, for example, didn't believe that his girl-friend wanted to be furiously pumped in the back seat of a car and that she gained as much satisfaction from such action as he did, he wouldn't push so hard for that sort of selfish sex.

When my wife and I are in the position and feeling very close, one of us is likely, spontaneously, to say, "I love you." It has a lot more than the I-love-you goodbye at the train station. Oh yes, and don't forget to call.

That's what makes it great. You have to be in love, you have to be reasonably happy, and then CAT works best.

RUTH
Wiping Out the Patriarchy

I've learned you have to be really open to appreciate the receiving part of the alignment. Trouble is, most of us aren't good at communi-cation. A committed relationship makes a difference. I've been talking to some young women who are starting to have sex for the first time and are interested in learning about the alignment. They realize they just can't drop one partner and find another one, and in the age of AIDS that's especially so.

There are so many assumptions about sex that aren't true—like it gets boring after you've been with the same partner for a long time. To experience *depth* with a person on a consistent basis you have to be willing to work on emotional blocks. A lot of people are into fantasy, just superficial sex. You can have an orgasm if you masturbate or from ordinary intercourse. Most anybody can come, but orgasm with the alignment transcends the ordinary kind.

Once I got into it, I was just totally open and relaxed, it was almost like floating. It felt very deep, and the connection with the other person was very deep. It was impossible for me to feel what I was feeling without my partner feeling the same thing. There was a sense of . . . presence. Having a simultaneous orgasm is not just mechanical, it's a oneness, just like total knowledge and understanding of each other.

Maybe I'm romanticizing the alignment, but having had the experience, I just can't play around anymore. It just doesn't work. On the other hand, there was a time . . . I don't quite understand ... when I could have the pleasure of alignment and then walk away from it. I'd had so much pain in my life that I did walk away from it, it would disarm me, scare me, and then I would do things to negate it. I guess I was still sort of enslaved by my past. No more, but it can happen.

I know it's jargon, but I see the alignment as empowering for young women because so many of them seem to think that, well, the boyfriend must know what to do. They've been taught that. It's like giving them permission to have their own kind of orgasm, the alignment seems like a natural thing for women compared to the friction of traditional intercourse. Friction does nothing for a woman, not enough, anyway. Some of these young women have no idea what I am talking about, and because they've had orgasms from masturbation they focus on *that* kind of release more in the relationship. You can have a clitoral orgasm that way, but it's pretty superficial, anyway, not at all like the complete orgasms in the alignment that involve the cervix and the uterus. It's something that you feel deeply in your body, whereas clitoral orgasm is, well, like a man's masturbatory ejaculation.

You could say the alignment is just about the most powerfully egalitarian thing that a man and woman can do. Women are *still* living under patriarchy, and patriarchy influences everything—how we think, how we behave, how we relate, how we talk with men. The alignment just wipes out all that. To use the current vernacular, it gives you a level playing field.

MIKE
Down With the Old—Up With the Alignment

Proper breathing creates a relaxed and comfortable feeling. It's the most obvious sign of how together you are. There are other layers, but breathing seems to be an obvious test of how connected or disconnected the movement is. I check how my partner is feeling that way.

Traditionally we've learned to use other sounds and signals as being the equivalent of "good," such as a woman writhing around. Breathing is really fine-tuning, taking an overwhelming situation and focusing it.

It would be interesting to know if, in fact, women are more prone to this kind of love making, low-keyed and sensual. All these centuries men have been sort of put on by the thrashing and screaming to please and appease their egos. It's a matter of maturity, too. It takes time to know someone well enough to risk not pushing the old classic buttons.

I find it a lot less distracting to be on top. My head and part of my shoulder are off. It's almost like being side-by-side, and at the same time being on top of each other for the movement itself. Whenever I get away from that position, it feels artificial. My wife encourages me to get on top because it's the most satisfying position for her as well.

I think the *intent* of the alignment is different. The traditional conquest aspect isn't there—or at least it certainly isn't as dominant. As far as the physical outcome, I would say orgasm lasts longer, even if it's measured in seconds.

MILES
Learning to Be a Rocker

Annette and I had dated off and on for several months. The sex had followed the tide of the relationship itself, which is to say, it alternated between blind ecstasy and rote indifference, with the occasional no go. In making love, she always responded best when things moved very slowly, when the foreplay was extended, when I kissed, fondled and caressed her body for an hour or more. Then, when I pulled out the baby oil lotion (a favorite), we would both instinctively explode (as if on cue!) into bang-up (no pun intended) intercourse. Conversely, the times that I pushed it were invariably the times that she simply shut down. When all moved well, she had no trouble coming during traditional intercourse or oral sex, very often several times.

It was one of those nights, one of those happy and uninhibited nights when, in the middle of a basic thrust (I was on top), she suddenly grabbed my hips and whispered to me, "No, don't ... slow down ... stop." At first, of course, I panicked, imagining that perhaps we were back in the "rushing it" category, that I'd made some wrong, horrifyingly anti-erotic maneuver that signalled to Annette—"system shut down."

Not the case! She grabbed me passionately, and as I looked at her, I could see that the expression on her face was not one of frustration, but of happiness and anticipation. She said, "Stop ... just rock, so slow, so slow ..." She grabbed me tightly, and then with her hands on my hips she guided the way she wanted me to go. She lifted me slightly higher so that my body was more acutely on top of hers. And as I tried to thrust (because I still didn't know exactly what she had in mind), she held me back. I was still inside her, but rather than pushing in and out, she led me into what I would call almost sliding my shaft along her clitoris in a slow, rocking, almost circular motion. I could see on her face that this was deeply erotic to her, that, compared with the look on her face just a few moments before (traditional style), she was in another zone. Her head arched back, her eyes closed tight, she whispered to just keep doing that, doing that.

In what seemed just a few seconds, she came. She came for what at the time felt like thirty or forty seconds, writhing and almost crying and even letting out a small yelp. Before she was always silent during sex, which I don't find arousing. I prefer a woman who makes noise, reacts. I think Annette saw sex as a solemn, secret pleasure shared by two, whereas I tend to see it as a kind of small celebration, a party. For my own part, I have to say that this first time, this rocking intercourse method didn't do much for me. I even had a bit of difficulty staying hard, since the friction wasn't there and since I wasn't certain where we were going. I overcame that and soon looked forward to the rocking because it gave her such obvious pleasure, as nothing else did: because even though I was hesitant about losing control the first time, I eventually came around to enjoying having her in control. It seemed in some ways more a *shared* experience, more purely conjugal in a way than just me thrusting away.

CONSTANCE
Laughing Out Loud

Most people had difficulty with the alignment at first: Who's holding back? Whose machismo is threatened? Who can't put out because that's not his or her role? In alignment you're either giving something that you weren't giving before and/or giving up something that you weren't giving up before.

Depending on what your particular problem is—whether it's risk-taking or vulnerability—people are pretty much locked into roles.

In the days when I was sleeping around, the man had his part and the woman had her part, and, pretty much, you didn't stray from that. That was "safe." In order to do the alignment you have to get *out* of the rut. The woman has to contribute her fifty percent. And the man has to allow her to—if you will—and see that as a positive thing.

All that couples need is *one* good experience. It could even happen by accident or by trust. For some women the challenge is contributing and not letting themselves be fucked. Or feeling, okay, so here I am, do me. For another kind of woman the challenge might be getting past all the political implications: "What do you mean he has to be on top?" Or, the woman might have to hold back, she might be contributing too much, and not letting him do *his* bit. Certain people feel more comfortable being the "fuck*ee*" and others being the "fuck*ers*." The roles are not, after all, unique to either sex.

For years I thought I was having orgasms,

but I wasn't. There was pleasurable sensation, certainly. Okay, maybe it was orgasm to the extent that I was capable of experiencing one. The alignment is how I know that there is more to orgasm. This is no fluke. This is a *real* revelation. The first time it ever worked for me and my husband, I laughed out loud—*from the tip of my toes to the top of my head.*

The thing about having this incredible orgasm on the alignment is that you realize that you can feel even more positive about your partner because this isn't something that somebody else *did* to you. You did this thing *together.* You don't think, this guy is *a great lover.* It's not just him—it's you, too! I think you feel better about the other person *because* it wasn't all him. Rather than hero-worship— or idolizing the other person—you're just grateful. Intercourse is more equitable.

Personally, I don't have this incredible libido. I would just as soon go for the big one. Once I've had that, I really don't have to do it again. Excuse the pun—it's anti-climactic. If the first orgasm is really good, I don't want to chance following up with something that is *less* good. But I'm not saying that if you have the stamina you couldn't do it again. I'm grateful for the first one—I'm not greedy. But if it's there for you, be happy and accept it.

SHEILA
Like Setting Up a Tent

The alignment solidified my relationship so much with my husband Ralph that to this day we've never really separated our lives. If I was to try it with another man, I wonder if I would then be able to let go of Ralph. That's how strong the dynamic is with the alignment. It's an integral part of the relationship.

We always thought that our marriage was a kind of healing, that whatever we didn't get from our parents, we brought to our own family. We were going to make up for everything that had been wrong in our childhoods. But it's not only that you have your own positive sexual experience; you *share* that with another person. And you can't do that with ordinary sex. And you can't be successful with the alignment unless you have these rather subtle feelings.

True, you can have so-called good sex without communication. In fact, regular sex was better if I didn't communicate. Talking about it lost something in the translation, everything was supposed to be spontaneous, wasn't it?

But talking seems to be an important part of the alignment. It's not staying mute to be "spontaneous." It's sort of like setting up a tent ... you hold this and I'll hold that and the tent gets assembled, so to speak.

The actual physical stimulation, as in masturbation, is intense, *especially* because you're sharing it with another person. That's the miracle and the risk of the alignment. There were lots of times when I was so excited about being alive and being who I was that it was almost impossible to show that level of excitement to another person in bed. It's something very private. I have all kinds of secrets. But to be able to open up sexually with another person in the alignment and know that he is feeling the same thing is just a wonderful experience.

I wasn't able to reach orgasm easily through intercourse before the alignment. They say women must be in love in order to focus and then achieve their orgasm. I'm forty-four now, but the big change in my life has been the alignment and what it has made possible. It has confirmed that golden oldie that the partners need to feel deeply about each other to achieve the fullest satisfaction in sex.

A FINAL WORD FROM DR. ARTHUR SCHOR

From 1971 through 1974 I was in psychotherapy. It was part of my training as a psychotherapist. My therapist/teacher/mentor had been a monk and brought a kind of spiritual and Eastern way of thinking to the abstractions of psychotherapy.

I had explored issues, often about relationships, and had the opportunity to question and challenge many culturally determined concepts or beliefs. In short, I had believed in cultural truths that limited my experiencing life, including sex.

While undergoing treatment, and not focusing on sexual issues much at all, my sex life began to alter. I'd say it went from normal excitement and satisfaction to something that seemed impossible.

During intercourse I had naturally begun to position myself differently. I was moving more slowly, less in-and-out motion, more a staying-in and upward pressure.

The new experiences included having a heightened sense of relaxation, blending, melting, connecting, timelessness and mindlessness.

Orgasms became naturally simultaneous during intercourse. Multiple orgasms were more frequent, the length of time of lovemaking became sweetly longer, and I began to stay awake and energetic after my orgasm.

I am now forty-seven-years old. I had been married, but for only four years, and have had several intimate relationships with women. A few of the women with whom I have had such intimacy were able to share this new sexual experience, as is the woman I am now with and plan to marry.

I believe that this analogy may serve to begin to understand the value and implications of the alignment:

Training wheels are to bicycling as the Coital Alignment Technique is to the new sex.

Training wheels allow an individual to practice and practice until the *natural* ability to balance is *incorporated*. Once incorporated, a person can then *always* balance a bicycle. Practice does not cause balancing, it provides an opportunity to achieve it. Although balancing a bicycle is natural, people are not able to achieve it without practice, and usually experience awkwardness when beginning. This occurs even after having watched many others bicycling.

The practicing of the CAT allows couples an access to this new sexual experience that, once achieved, becomes incorporated. The "new sex" is natural. It is difficult to achieve without practice and undergoing some awkwardness. But the payoff is more than appropriate compensation.

Appendix

The following tables are based on data from Edward Eichel's study in the Human Sexuality Program at New York University validating and assessing the effectiveness of the Coital Alignment Technique. The study compares, by percentages, an experimental-research group of twenty-one men and twenty-two women trained in the CAT technique and a control group of twenty-one men and twenty-two women who were not so trained. The data measure different factors of technique and response and summarize participants' opinions about the implications. The data compare pre- and post-training experiences of the men and women who first experimented with the CAT technique. Percentage tables are headed by questions from the questionnaire that was used in the NYU study.

THE PERFECT FIT

Did you fantasize less during intercourse in alignment?

Frequency	TRAINED Males	UNTRAINED Females
Very much	42.9%	31.8%
Somewhat	33.3%	13.6%
Not at all	—	13.6%
Don't fantasize during intercourse	23.8%	40.9%

Was orgasm in sexual intercourse more intense than orgasm with masturbation?

Frequency	TRAINED Males/Females	UNTRAINED Males/Females
Very much	67.4%	44.2%
Somewhat	11.6%	27.9%
Not at all	9.3%	20.9%
Don't masturbate to orgasm	11.6%	7.0%

Did alignment increase your desire to have sex more frequently?

Frequency	TRAINED Males	TRAINED Females
Very much	33.3%	40.9%
Somewhat	28.5%	22.7%
Not at all	38.1%	36.4%

Appendix

Which position do you prefer for sexual intercourse?

Position	TRAINED Females	UNTRAINED Females
Man-above	72.7%	27.3%
Woman-above	9.1%	31.8%
Side-by-side	9.1%	18.2%
Rear entry	—	13.6%
Other	9.1%	9.1%

Which position do you prefer for orgasm?

Position	TRAINED Females	UNTRAINED Females
Man-above	63.6%	18.2%
Woman-above	22.7%	40.9%
Side-by-side	4.5%	4.5%
Rear entry	4.5%	9.1%
Other	4.5%	18.2%
Do not reach orgasm in intercourse	—	9.1%

THE PERFECT FIT

Can you reach orgasm in the man-above position without manual stimulation?

Frequency	TRAINED Females	UNTRAINED Females
Always/Almost Always	31.8%	13.6%
Often	45.5%	13.6%
Sometimes	22.7%	22.7%
Rarely	—	31.8%
Never	—	9.1%
Do not try to reach orgasm in this position	—	9.1%

Frequency of female orgasm in the man-above position before and after learning alignment

Frequency	Before training	After training
Always/Almost always	4.5%	50.0%
Often	18.2%	27.3%
Sometimes	31.8%	13.6%
Rarely	31.8%	9.1%
Never	13.6%	—

Appendix

How often have you and your partner reached orgasm at about the same time in the man-above position?

Frequency	TRAINED Females	UNTRAINED Females
Always/Almost Always	18.2%	—
Often	18.2%	9.1%
Sometimes	36.4%	13.6%
Rarely	27.3%	45.5%
Never	—	22.7%
Don't know	—	—
Do not reach orgasm in this position	—	9.1%
Partner doesn't reach orgasm in this position	—	—

Note: Answers based on respondents' past and/or present experience.

THE PERFECT FIT

How often have you and your partner reached orgasm at about the same time in the man-above position?

Frequency	TRAINED Males	UNTRAINED Males
Always/Almost Always	14.3%	—
Often	33.3%	9.5%
Sometimes	28.6%	47.6%
Rarely	23.8%	19.0%
Never	—	19.9%
Don't know	—	—
Do not reach orgasm in this position	—	—
Partner doesn't reach orgasm in this position	—	4.8%

Note: Answers based on respondents' past and/or present experience.

Frequency of simultaneous orgasm in females in man-above before and after learning alignment?

Frequency	Before Training	After Training
Always/Almost Always	—	36.4%
Often	4.5%	13.6%
Sometimes	18.2%	31.8%
Rarely	59.1%	18.2%
Never	18.2%	—

Appendix

Frequency of simultaneous orgasm in males in man-above before and after learning alignment?

Frequency	TRAINED Males/Females	UNTRAINED Males/Females
Always/Almost Always	4.8%	38.1%
Often	4.8%	19.0%
Sometimes	52.4%	33.3%
Rarely	23.8%	9.5%
Never	14.3%	—

Index

Index